FIVE DIFFERENT BOOKS IN ONE
COLOR-CODED
FOR YOUR CONVENIENCE

- SUPERMARKET-SHOPPING GUIDE—with calorie counter
- EASY-DOES-IT WEIGHT LOSS PLAN—complete with calorie-activity chart
- LOW-FAT-COOKING GUIDE—with delicious recipes, spice-magic tables, and calorie counts
- A GUIDE TO DINING OUT—breakfast, lunch, and dinner menus for Italian, French, and Greek restaurants and delicatessens *PLUS*
  A COMPLETE GUIDE TO FAST-FOOD RESTAURANTS—with item-by-item calorie, cholesterol, and fat counts for the major fast-food chains
- HEALTH GUIDE—a doctor answers your questions about diet and heart disease

Keep the life-saving facts at your fingertips for fast, easy instant reference with
THE DELL COLOR-CODED LOW-FAT-LIVING GUIDE.

THE DELL COLOR-CODED LOW-FAT-LIVING GUIDE

Janet James and Lois Goulder

A DELL BOOK

Published by
Dell Publishing Co., Inc.
1 Dag Hammarskjold Plaza
New York, New York 10017

Dell ® TM 681510, Dell Publishing Co., Inc.

ISBN: 0-440-17621-2

Printed in the United States of America

First printing—June 1980

TABLE OF CONTENTS

6

PART I

THE FAT FACTS OF LIFE: HEART ATTACK IS THE NATION'S NUMBER ONE KILLER.

The latest figures from the U.S. Department of Health, Education and Welfare report that 640,000 people died from heart attacks in 1977.*

You can reduce your risk of heart attack. You may save your own life by:

Eating foods with less saturated fat
Eating foods with less cholesterol

Three leading national health authorities make these recommendations to consume less saturated fat and cholesterol:

The American Heart Association
The U.S. Senate Select Committee on Nutrition and Human Needs
The Inter-Society Commission for Heart Disease Resources

Their advice is based on strong evidence that a diet high in saturated fat/cholesterol is linked to a high incidence of coronary heart disease.

---

*Since the U.S. Government accumulates data over a three-year period before publication, the 1977 statistics are the most current available.

SATURATED FAT and CHOLESTEROL are the names for two types of fat found in foods. There is also a third kind of fat in foods which is called POLYUNSATURATED FAT.

You may *increase* your risk of coronary heart disease if you eat foods with too much saturated fat and cholesterol; on the other hand, you may *decrease* your risk of coronary heart disease if you eat foods with polyunsaturated fat.

Following is an explanation of the three types of fats in foods:

SATURATED FAT is a type of fat found in foods from animal sources such as meats and dairy products. Saturated fat is also found in some foods from vegetable sources, such as coconut oil, palm oil, and cocoa butter.

CHOLESTEROL is another type of fat found *ONLY* in foods from animal sources, such as meats and dairy products.

POLYUNSATURATED FATS are found mainly in foods from vegetable sources. They are oils (liquid at room temperature) such as corn, safflower, sesame, soybean, sunflower, peanut, and cottonseed.

The U.S. Senate Select Committee on Nutrition and Human Needs heard health and nutrition experts from all over the country testify that *Americans eat too much fat!* In their committee report, *Dietary Goals for the United States*, they made the following recommendations concerning fat in the daily American diet:

1. Americans should REDUCE "overall fat consumption" from 40% to 30% of energy intake (calories).
2. Americans should REDUCE saturated fat consumption from 16% to 10% of energy intake.

3. Americans should REDUCE cholesterol consumption from 600 milligrams (mgs.) to 300 milligrams (mgs.).
4. Americans should INCREASE polyunsaturated fat consumption from 7% to 10% of energy intake.

The *Dietary Goals* compares:

WHAT AMERICANS NOW EAT (IN RED) with WHAT AMERICANS SHOULD EAT (IN GREEN).

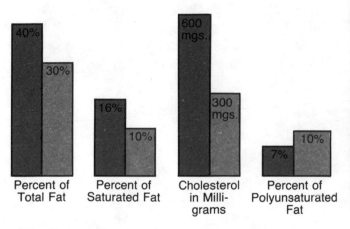

| Percent of Total Fat | Percent of Saturated Fat | Cholesterol in Milligrams | Percent of Polyunsaturated Fat |

The *Dietary Goals* recommends that we SHOULD EAT:

¼ LESS TOTAL FAT
⅓ LESS SATURATED FAT
½ LESS CHOLESTEROL
⅓ MORE POLYUNSATURATED FAT

To reduce the risk of coronary heart disease, therefore, we should consume LESS SATURATED FAT AND CHOLESTEROL, and consume more polyunsaturated fat.

The *Dietary Goals* points out that for anyone who is overweight, "the best protection against heart disease is weight reduction." The American Heart Association supports this view and states:

Avoidance of obesity, early in life, or a supervised weight reduction for those above their ideal body weight, is strongly recommended.

Because of this relationship between obesity (overweight) and heart disease, a special section, "Enjoy Losing Weight," is included in this LOW-FAT-LIVING GUIDE. To help you shop for foods low in calories, a "CALORIE COUNTER" begins on page 92.

PART II

THE COLOR CODE IS THE KEY

To help you follow these recommendations for better health, THE LOW-FAT-LIVING GUIDE uses a color code which is keyed to the colors of a traffic signal:

GREEN IS GO—FOR BETTER HEALTH.

FOODS LOW IN SATURATED FAT ARE IN GREEN.

FOODS HIGH IN POLYUNSATURATED FAT ARE IN GREEN.

FOODS LOW IN CHOLESTEROL ARE IN GREEN.

YELLOW IS CAUTION.

FOODS MODERATE IN SATURATED FAT ARE IN YELLOW.

FOODS MODERATE IN CHOLESTEROL ARE IN YELLOW.

RED IS STOP—DANGER.

FOODS HIGH IN SATURATED FAT WITH HIGH OR MODERATE CHOLESTEROL ARE IN RED.

FOODS HIGH IN CHOLESTEROL ONLY ARE IN RED.

The color code enables you to see at a glance what foods you should eat and what foods you should avoid.

The Dell Color-Coded Low-Fat-Living Guide is really five guides in one:

1. Supermarket-shopping guide
2. Guide to losing weight (with Calorie-Activity Chart)
3. Cooking guide: low-fat recipes
4. Dining-out guide, including fast-food restaurants
5. Health guide: A doctor answers questions on diet and heart disease.

You will find this color-coded guide of invaluable help if you want to improve your health by following the Senate Committee's advice to reduce the amount of saturated fat, cholesterol, and calories you consume daily.

A companion guide to better health, written by the same authors, is *The Dell Color-Coded Low-Salt-Living Guide* which will help you to reduce the amount of salt/sodium in your diet. Special features include: the low-salt supermarket-shopping guide; exclusive low-sodium recipes (which are also low in fat); low-sodium guide for over-the-counter drugs; dining-out guide (including fast-food restaurants); and medical information on diet and high blood pressure. In both of these books the color code will brighten your way to healthier eating.

PART III

THE COLOR-CODED SUPERMARKET-SHOPPING GUIDE

HOW TO USE THIS SUPERMARKET GUIDE

AT HOME
to plan your meals low in saturated fat—
low in cholesterol

AT THE SUPERMARKET
to choose foods low in
saturated fat—low in cholesterol

WHEN CONSULTING WITH YOUR
DOCTOR OR DIETITIAN
if you are on a special diet.

This Shopping Guide will lead you through the supermarket, with a separate color-coded page for each department. On each page the foods are classified, by color, according to the saturated fat/cholesterol content of each food listed.

To make your choices, consult the Table of Contents at the front of the book for the page of the Supermarket Guide which lists the foods in that particular department.

THE COLOR CODE MAKES IT EASY TO CHOOSE:

YOU CAN BUY
The foods listed in GREEN:
Low in saturated fat
Low in cholesterol
High in polyunsaturated fat (oils)

YOU CAN BUY WITH CAUTION
The foods listed in YELLOW:
Moderate in saturated fat
Moderate in cholesterol

DON'T BUY
The foods listed in RED:
High in saturated fat with high or moderate cholesterol
High in cholesterol only

The color code will help you make healthier food choices at the supermarket. The foods are *color-coded within each department of the supermarket*, according to their relative content of saturated fat / cholesterol.

For example, if you are shopping for dairy products, turn to page 24 of this Guide for the Dairy Department.

Which milk product should you buy—buttermilk or whole milk? The color code immediately makes it clear. You should buy buttermilk listed in GREEN, rather than WHOLE MILK listed in RED

You will note that buttermilk and whole milk are listed in 1 cup (8 ounce) servings, considered to be the *usual serving* size. The Calorie Counter, beginning on page 92, lists all foods according to the amount of calories found in a usual serving of a particular food. The color code applies *only* to the serving size listed in the Calorie Counter.

The Calorie Counter is organized, like the Shopping Guide, according to each department of the supermarket. Each food is coded in the same color as the Supermarket Shopping Guide.

This Shopping Guide includes only those foods for which authoritative data on saturated fat and cholesterol are available. The sources of this data are listed in the Bibliography on pages 124 and 125. Some figures on fat content and calories were obtained from individual food manufacturers and are designated with an asterisk (*) in the Calorie Counter.

CHOOSE YOUR FOODS BY COLOR

Read across these pages to find the fat content of the following foods, and the department and page number where they are listed in the Supermarket **SHOPPING GUIDE**.

ALL FRESH FRUITS AND VEGETABLES
MOST CEREALS
FLOUR

FRESH MEATS: fat-trimmed*, lean, low-marbled* beef, lamb, pork, veal

POULTRY: chicken, turkey (no skin)

FRESH FISH: some fresh shellfish (crab, clams, lobster, oysters, scallops)

FROZEN FISH: frozen crab

DAIRY PRODUCTS: skim-milk products
1% or less milkfat products
2% cottage cheese

FATS: vegetable oils: safflower, sunflower, corn, soybean, sesame, peanut, cottonseed

FATS: polyunsaturated margarines

SEEDS AND NUTS

---

*See page 21 for explanation of "fat-trimmed" and "marbling."

INDEX TO SUPERMARKET FOOD

FAT CONTENT	SUPERMARKET DEPARTMENT	PAGE NUMBER
Low saturated fat No cholesterol	Produce	20
	Cereals	26
	Baking aids	28
Low saturated fat	Meats	21
	Poultry	21
Low cholesterol	Fish	21
	Frozen Foods	25
	Dairy Products	24
Low saturated fat	Oils	30
High polyunsaturated Fat No cholesterol	Dairy	24
	Produce	20
	Snacks	34

MEATS: fat-trimmed*, medium fat, medium marbled* beef, lamb, pork, veal

FRESH SHRIMP
FROZEN SHRIMP
CANNED SARDINES

DAIRY PRODUCTS: 2% milkfat products
4% creamed cottage cheese, some cheese

"NATURAL" CEREALS

FATS: vegetable shortening

VEGETABLE OIL: olive oil

MEATS: untrimmed, highly marbled* beef, lamb, pork, veal

DAIRY PRODUCTS: whole milk, butter, some cheese

ICE CREAM

EGG YOLK

ORGAN MEATS: brains, hearts, livers, kidneys, sweetbreads

*See page 21 for explanation of "fat-trimmed" and "marbling."

FAT CONTENT	DEPARTMENT	PAGE
Moderate saturated fat	Meats	22
Moderate cholesterol	Fish	22
	Frozen foods	25
	Canned foods	27
	Dairy	24
Moderate saturated fat	Cereals	26
No cholesterol	Baking aids	28
Low saturated fat Low polyunsaturated fat No cholesterol	Oils	30

High saturated fat	Meats	23
Moderate cholesterol	Dairy	24
	Ice Cream	33
High cholesterol only	Dairy	24
	Meats	23

DEPARTMENTS OF THE SUPERMARKET
FRESH PRODUCE

ALL FRESH FRUITS
(except coconut)

ALL DRIED FRUITS

FRESH ORANGE JUICE

FRESH GRAPEFRUIT JUICE

ALL FRESH VEGETABLES

See the Flavor-Magic Chart on pages
54 and 55 for new ways to season
vegetables.

ALL NUTS

FRESH COCONUT

FRESH MEATS, POULTRY, FISH—
PROCESSED MEATS

Lean meats are fat-trimmed and low-marbled.

"FAT-TRIMMED" means *ALL* the visible fat has been cut from the meat before cooking.

"MARBLING" refers to the streaks of fat that run *through* the meat. Choose *low-marbled* meat which has fewer streaks of fat.

BEEF: fat-trimmed, low-marbled round, rump, flank, chuck (arm), tenderloin, sirloin, plate (short ribs)

LAMB: fat-trimmed, low-marbled leg, loin, rib, shoulder

PORK: fat-trimmed, low-marbled fresh or smoked ham

VEAL: fat-trimmed all cuts (except veal breast)

POULTRY: without skin chicken, turkey

FISH: all kinds of fresh fish some shellfish: clams, crab, lobster, oysters, and scallops

PROCESSED MEATS—*only* those listed below; meats listed below are similar in fat content and calories to other meats listed in green:

LUNCHEON MEATS: dried beef, jellied corned beef, honey loaf, lean pastrami

PRESSED MEATS: chicken, turkey, corned beef, chip

SAUERKRAUT

BEEF: low to medium-marbled, fat-trimmed
  LOIN: porterhouse, T-bone

  GROUND BEEF is classified by fat content:

  GROUND ROUND: Fat cannot exceed 15%
  GROUND CHUCK: Fat cannot exceed 20%
  GROUND MEAT OR COMMERCIAL
  HAMBURGER: Fat cannot exceed 30%

Ground beef with lower fat content is more desirable for a diet low in saturated fat and cholesterol.

PORK: fat-trimmed

  BOSTON BUTT, CANADIAN BACON, PICNIC

FRESH SHRIMP

PROCESSED MEATS—*only* those listed below; meats listed below are similar in fat content and calories to other meats listed in yellow:

LUNCHEON MEATS: barbecue beef, Lebanon bologna, Dutch loaf, picnic loaf, olive loaf, pickle pimiento loaf, boiled ham

BEEF: fat not trimmed, highly marbled

rib roast, club, and rib steaks,
all other untrimmed beef cuts,
corned beef (brisket)
commercial hamburger

LAMB:

breast

PORK:

spareribs, loin and loin chops, canned
ham, bacon

VEAL:

breast

POULTRY:
duck, goose

PROCESSED MEATS:
any luncheon meats not listed in green
or yellow, as well as frankfurters, liverwurst, sausages

ORGAN MEATS:
all brains, hearts, kidneys, livers,
sweetbreads

LARD

DAIRY AND REFRIGERATED PRODUCTS

MILK: skim milk or low-fat milk, 1% fat
        buttermilk, cultured
        chocolate milk from low-fat, 1% fat

CHEESE: cottage cheese (dry cottage cheese,
          low-fat, 1% or 2% fat)
          processed skim milk cheese spread

MARGARINE (See page 44)

WHIPPED CREAM TOPPING (PRESSURIZED)
SMOKED SALMON   PICKLED HERRING
HORSERADISH   DILL PICKLES

MILK: low-fat milk, 2% fat
        chocolate milk from low-fat, 2% fat
        low-fat yogurt, 2% (plain and fruit-flavored)

CREAM: coffee cream, half-and-half, sour
         cream, whipping cream

CHEESE: Mozzarella (low moisture, part-skim),
          Ricotta (part-skim), Neufchatel, Par-
          mesan, creamed cottage cheese,
          4% milk-fat

EGG YOLK—A CONCENTRATED SOURCE OF
          CHOLESTEROL

BUTTER   IMITATION SOUR CREAM

MILK: whole milk, eggnog
        chocolate milk from whole milk

CHEESE: all except those listed in yellow or
          green
          creamed cottage cheese, 6% milk-fat

REFRIGERATED COOKIE DOUGH

FROZEN FOODS

ALL FROZEN FRUITS—ALL FROZEN JUICES

PLAIN, UNCOOKED FROZEN FISH

PLAIN, FROZEN CRAB

FROZEN POULTRY

FROZEN VEGETABLES: plain, sugar-glazed, and oriental

FROZEN EGG SUBSTITUTES

FROZEN WAFFLES (plain)

FROZEN ROLLS: Parkerhouse, poppy seed, sesame seed

FROZEN COFFEE WHITENER (non-dairy)

FROZEN DESSERT TOPPING (non-dairy), pressurized, and semi-solid

---

FROZEN TURKEY, butter-basted

PLAIN FROZEN SHRIMP (raw or precooked)

FROZEN MUFFINS   FROZEN EGG WAFFLES
FRENCH FRIED POTATOES

There is a wide variation in the saturated fat/cholesterol contents of frozen foods among different manufacturers. These include main course "TV" dinners, vegetables with sauces, pot pies, and prepared fish and shellfish products.

BREADED OR COATED FROZEN VEGETABLES

FROZEN FRIED FISH   FROZEN FRUIT AND
FROZEN   CAKES   CREAM   PIES
FROZEN PIZZA
FROZEN DOUGHNUTS
FROZEN CROISSANTS (BUTTER ROLLS)

CEREALS AND TOASTER PASTRIES

Cereals vary widely in calorie contents. Check the Calorie Counter on pages 103, 104, and 105 for calories on individual cereals.

ALL HOT CEREALS (served with skim milk)

MOST READY-TO-EAT CEREALS (served with skim milk)

WHEAT GERM

CORNMEAL

"NATURAL CEREALS" often contain COCO-NUT and/or COCONUT OIL or PALM OIL, which are highly saturated vegetable fats.

TOASTER PASTRIES

HOT AND READY-TO-EAT CEREALS
(served with whole milk)

BREAKFAST BARS

CANNED FOODS
FRUITS AND JUICES, VEGETABLES, SOUPS, FISH, MEATS, READY-TO-SERVE, CHINESE FOODS

ALL CANNED FRUITS AND FRUIT JUICES

ALL CANNED VEGETABLES AND VEGETABLE JUICES

CANNED FISH: CRAB, SALMON, AND TUNA

CANNED SOUPS PREPARED WITH WATER, DEHYDRATED SOUPS, BOUILLON CUBES

CANNED SPAGHETTI IN TOMATO SAUCE (WITH CHEESE)

CANNED BAKED BEANS IN TOMATO SAUCE

CANNED PORK AND BEANS

CHINESE DINNERS   SOY SAUCE

CANNED CREAM SOUPS prepared with low-fat milk

CANNED CHEESE SOUP prepared with low-fat milk

CANNED SPAGHETTI AND MEATBALLS

CANNED MACARONI AND CHEESE

CANNED SARDINES   CANNED SHRIMP

CANNED VIENNA SAUSAGE

CANNED VEGETABLE AND BEEF STEW

CANNED BEANS AND FRANKS

CANNED CHILI CON CARNE

CANNED PORK (chopped, spiced/unspiced)
CANNED PORK SAUSAGE (patties)

CAKE AND PIE MIXES, DESSERTS, BAKING AIDS

ALL FLOURS   ALL SUGARS
                 BAKING SODA
BAKING POWDER   CORNSTARCH
           PANCAKE SYRUP
GELATINS   DRY TAPIOCA
MAPLE SYRUP   MOLASSES
NONFAT DRY MILK, EVAPORATED SKIM MILK
                         (canned)
ANGEL-FOOD CAKE MIX
"LIGHT" FROSTING MIX
GRAHAM-CRACKER CRUMBS FOR PIECRUSTS
POWDERED DESSERT TOPPING (NONDAIRY)
FLAVORINGS AND LIQUEUR EXTRACTS
PUDDING MIXES PREPARED WITH SKIM MILK

VEGETABLE SHORTENING (solid)
CAKE FROSTING MIXES
PUDDING MIXES PREPARED WITH WHOLE
   MILK
EVAPORATED WHOLE MILK (canned)

DRY MIXES FOR BISCUITS, CAKES, MUF-
   FINS, PANCAKES, AND WAFFLES
Preferred mixes DO NOT INCLUDE EGG YOLKS
AND/OR SHORTENING. USE "egg substitutes"
or two egg whites INSTEAD OF one whole
egg. Use skim or nonfat dry milk INSTEAD OF
whole milk.

CHOCOLATE (bitter, baking, semisweet)
SWEETENED CONDENSED MILK (canned)
SHREDDED COCONUT   PIECRUST MIX

SPAGHETTI, NOODLES, RICE, BEANS, SAUCES

RICE (white, brown, and instant)

DRY MACARONI AND SPAGHETTI
DRY NOODLES

DRIED BEANS, LENTILS, AND PEAS

TOMATO PASTE, PUREE, SAUCE

MEATLESS SPAGHETTI SAUCE (bottled)

DRY GRAVY MIXES (prepared with water)

PIZZA CRUST MIX   CHEESE PIZZA MIX

SPAGHETTI SAUCE WITH MEAT (bottled)

DEHYDRATED POTATOES
Prepared with skim milk and margarine instead of whole milk and butter

---

PIZZA MIXES WITH MEAT

DRY GRAVY MIXES (prepared with milk)

MACARONI AND NOODLE "MAIN-DISH DINNERS"
The saturated fat/cholesterol content of macaroni and noodle dinners is increased when ground meat is added. Use the guidelines on page 22 to select ground meat with lower fat content.

SALAD DRESSINGS, OLIVES, PICKLES, OILS

ALL VEGETABLE OILS (except olive oil)
(See page 39 for information on fat content of vegetable oils)

PACKAGED SALAD DRESSING MIXES (dry)
(prepared with vegetable oils listed above or buttermilk)

BOTTLED SALAD DRESSINGS*

CHILI SAUCE	KETCHUP
PICKLES	PICKLE RELISH
ALL VINEGARS	PREPARED MUSTARD
IMITATION BACON BITS	
WORCESTERSHIRE SAUCE	BARBECUE SAUCE

---

*BOTTLED SALAD DRESSINGS: Some salad dressings may have small amounts of cholesterol in the added cheese, eggs, or sour cream.

MAYONNAISE	MAYONNAISE-TYPE DRESSING
OLIVES (green and ripe)	OLIVE OIL

HERBS AND SPICES

ALLSPICE, BASIL, BACON BITS (imitation), BAY LEAF, CARAWAY SEED, CARDAMOM, CELERY SALT, CELERY SEED, CHERVIL, CHILI POWDER, CINNAMON, CLOVES, CUMIN, CURRY POWDER, DILL SEED AND WEED, FENNEL, GARLIC POWDER, GARLIC SALT, GINGER, MACE, MARJORAM, MONOSODIUM GLUTAMATE (MSG), DRY MUSTARD, NUTMEG, ONION POWDER, ONION SALT, OREGANO, PAPRIKA, PARSLEY FLAKES, PEPPER (BLACK, CAYENNE, WHITE), POPPY SEED, POULTRY SEASONING, PUMPKIN-PIE SPICE, ROSEMARY, SAFFRON, SAGE, SAVORY, SESAME SEED, TARRAGON, THYME

Use the "Flavor-Magic" chart on pages 54 and 55 for new ways to season foods low in saturated fat/cholesterol. The suggested seasonings are salt free, and especially helpful to anyone on a sodium-restricted diet.

PACKAGED BAKERY: BREAD, ROLLS, CAKES AND PIES—COOKIES, AND CRACKERS

BREADS:
cracked wheat   pumpernickel
French or Vienna   raisin
Italian   rye
pita   white enriched
                       whole wheat

CRACKERS: graham crackers, matzos, melba toast, saltines, soda crackers, rye wafers, zwieback

ENGLISH MUFFINS   BREAD STICKS

COOKIES: fig bars, gingersnaps, lady fingers, vanilla wafers

ROLLS: brown and serve, cloverleaf, frankfurter, hamburger, and Kaiser

CORN FLAKE CRUMBS   BREAD CRUMBS
BREAD STUFFING, DRY
HERB-SEASONED CROUTONS

Many packaged bakery foods contain coconut and palm oils, which are highly saturated vegetable fats. See pages 35–40 for information on fat content of bakery products.

ALL COOKIES AND CRACKERS NOT LISTED IN GREEN

CAKES   CUPCAKES   DOUGHNUTS   PIES

DANISH PASTRY   CHEESE CRACKERS

JELLIES, CANDY, ICE CREAM, SYRUPS

ALL JELLIES, JAMS, MARMALADES

HONEY   MARSHMALLOWS

SHERBET   PEANUT BUTTER

GUM DROPS, HARD CANDY, CREAM MINTS,
CANDY CORN, BUTTERSCOTCH, JELLY
BEANS

CANNED CHOCOLATE SYRUP (thin-type)

ICE MILK

CARAMEL CANDY (plain)

ALL CHOCOLATE CANDY
  (milk and semisweet)

ICE CREAM

CHOCOLATE SYRUP (fudge-type)

BUTTERSCOTCH SAUCE

SNACKS	BEVERAGES
PRETZELS	COFFEE
ALL NUTS	TEA
CARAMEL CORN	SOFT DRINKS
POPCORN	WINE, BEER
UNPOPPED CORN (prepared with oils listed in green on page 39)	COCOA (dry powder)
	CHOCOLATE,
PEANUTS	STRAW-BERRY INSTANT DRINK MIX*
SOY NUTS	COFFEE WHITENER (powdered, non-dairy)
SUNFLOWER SEEDS	

Many snack foods contain coconut and/or palm oil, highly saturated vegetable fats.

*Cocoa, chocolate, or strawberry instant mixes should be prepared with skim milk, low-fat milk, or nonfat dry milk.

CORN CHIPS
POTATO CHIPS

CHEESES

FOOD LABELING: WHAT'S IN THE FOODS WE EAT?

WE AMERICANS HAVE A RIGHT TO KNOW WHAT'S IN THE FOODS WE EAT!

And we want that information printed clearly on the product label.

This message from consumers came across loud and clear to three government agencies. In 1978 the Food and Drug Administration, the U.S. Department of Agriculture, and the Federal Trade Commission held nationwide hearings in five U.S. cities to listen to the public voice their concerns about food labeling.

Anyone on a diet low in saturated fat and cholesterol needs labels which specifically list the *kinds* of fats contained in a product, and the specific *amounts* of those fats.

The nutrition information on food labels already includes total fat content (in grams), but a consumer has no way of knowing how much is saturated, and how much is polyunsaturated. Only a few products such as margarines, peanut butter, and mayonnaise identify the fat content as saturated and polyunsaturated fats.

Fat may be identified on a label as "shortening"—either animal or vegetable.

What does "animal shortening" mean?

It means fats from animals—beef fat or beef tallow, butter, chicken fat, and lard.

It is important that the label contain this information because these are SATURATED FATS. They all CONTAIN CHOLESTEROL, and should be avoided.

What does "vegetable shortening" mean on a label?

It could mean SATURATED FATS (COCONUT OIL, PALM OIL, AND COCOA BUTTER). Products containing these ingredients should be avoided.

It could also mean POLYUNSATURATED FATS. These are more desirable for anyone on a diet low in saturated fat/cholesterol.

Cookie and cracker labels use the terms "animal and vegetable shortening." Here's how a typical label might read:

> Animal or vegetable shortening containing one or more of the following: partially hydrogenated soybean oil, cottonseed oil and/or palm oil, coconut oil, lard.

This label is totally inadequate because it does not tell you if the product contains just one or ALL of the fats listed. It also doesn't give you any idea of what quantity there is of any one or all of the fats.

The label uses the term "hydrogenated," which adds to the confusion. Hydrogenation is a special process which makes vegetable oils hard at room temperature. This decreases the amount of polyunsaturates in the oil. A "hydrogenated" oil, therefore, is less desirable for a low-fat diet than a polyunsaturated oil.

Any product with a label similar to the one just mentioned probably does contain coconut oil, palm oil, and/or lard—ALL SATURATED FATS. So leave it on the supermarket shelf!

If a product label lists "animal shortening," then you know it contains cholesterol. A few products already list cholesterol content in milligrams (mgs.), both per serving and per hundred grams. Since most products do not yet list cholesterol content, see pages 41–43 for information on the cholesterol content of some common foods.

Perhaps the single most important guideline to remember when reading labels is: *A FOOD LABEL LISTS INGREDIENTS IN ORDER OF QUANTITY.* The first ingredient is largest in quantity, and the rest follow in diminishing order.

Anyone counting calories should know that most products include the number of calories per serving in the nutrition information on the label.

Many products use the word *Natural* on the package. Most people believe that a product labeled "natural" is good for one's health. This is not always true. Just read the label on a "natural" cereal. Note the number of grams of fat: from four to six grams, depending on the brand. Read the ingredient list, which includes both coconut and coconut oil among the first ingredients.

Compare the fat content of the "natural" cereal with plain, old-fashioned corn flakes. Note the number of grams of fat: zero. *Then decide which cereal you should choose for breakfast.*

Products with labels which state "No Cholesterol" may still contain some highly saturated vegetable fats—coconut oil, palm oil, and cocoa butter.

The joint efforts of consumer groups and government agencies should lead to better labeling of the fat content of foods in the future. Until then, use the following pages to help you identify the fats in foods:

FAT CONTENT OF COMMON OILS
(in grams per 100 grams of fat)

The following vegetable oils are listed in order of saturation, from the lowest to the highest.

CHOOSE THE VEGETABLE OILS WITH HIGHER RATIOS OF POLYUNSATURATES TO SATURATES (P/S RATIO). Avoid the oils listed in red—coconut oil, palm oil, and cocoa butter.

VEGETABLE OILS	Polyun-saturates	Saturates	Poly/Sat Ratio* P/S
Safflower	74	9	8:1
Sunflower	64	10	6:1
Corn	58	13	5:1
Soybean	58	15	4:1
Sesame	41	15	3:1
Soybean and Cottonseed	48	18	3:1
Soybean, hydrogenated	37	15	2:1
Cottonseed	51	26	2:1
Peanut	30	19	2:1
Olive	9	14	<1:1 *
PALM	9	48	**
COCOA BUTTER	3	60	**
COCONUT	2	86	**

*Ratio Symbol: <—less than
**These are very high in saturates.

"References for Fat Composition of Foods—Plant Products and Animal Products." *Journal of the American Dietetic Association*, Series 1975, 1976, 1977, 1978

FAT CONTENT OF ANIMAL FATS

"Animal shortening" is listed among the ingredients on many products, including cookies, crackers, bakery products, soups, snacks, and frozen dinners.

Listed below are the animal fats contained in foods, in increasing order of saturation. These animal fats are very high in saturates.

ANIMAL FAT	Polyun-saturates	Saturates
Chicken fat	18	33
Lard	12	40
Beef tallow	4	48
Butter	3	50

CHOLESTEROL CONTENT OF FOODS
(in milligrams)

The foods listed on the following three pages all contain cholesterol. Those color coded in red have the highest content of cholesterol.

FOOD	SERVING SIZE	CHOLESTEROL CONTENT (mgs.)
Meats: (cooked, lean, fat-trimmed)		
Beef	4 oz.	104
Lamb	4 oz.	113
Pork	4 oz.	100
Veal	4 oz.	112
Poultry: (without skin, cooked)		
Chicken, breast meat only	4 oz.	89
Chicken, drumstick meat only	4 oz.	104
Turkey, light meat	4 oz.	87
Turkey, dark meat	4 oz.	115
Organ Meats: (cooked)		
Kidneys, all kinds	4 oz.	908
Liver (beef, calf, hog, lamb)	1 slice (3 oz.)	372
Chicken liver	3 small	561
Fish and Shellfish: (cooked)		
Halibut	4 oz.	68
Lobster, meat only	4 oz.	96
Salmon, fresh	4 oz.	46
Salmon, canned	4 oz.	40

Sardines, canned	3¾ oz. can	127
Scallops	4 oz.	60
Shrimp, canned	20 small	51
Tuna, canned in water	3½ oz. can	62
Crab, canned, meat only	½ cup	81

Dairy Products:

Butter, stick	1 Tbs.	35
Margarine (all vegetable)	1 Tbs.	0

Milk:

Buttermilk	1 cup	5
Whole milk	1 cup	34
Low-fat 1%	1 cup	14
Low-fat 2%	1 cup	22
Skim	1 cup	5
Chocolate flavor, 2% fat	1 cup	20

Cream:

Half-and-half	1 Tbs.	6
Light coffee	1 Tbs.	10
Sour cream	1 Tbs.	8
Whipped topping (pressurized)	1 Tbs.	3
Whipping cream, heavy	1 Tbs.	20

One Egg or One Egg Yolk: 250

Cheese: (natural and processed)

American, pasteurized	1 oz.	25
Blue	1 oz.	24
Brick	1 oz.	25
Camembert	1 oz.	26
Cheddar	1 oz.	28
Colby	1 oz.	27

Cottage cheese, creamed

1% fat	½ cup	12
4% fat	½ cup	24
uncreamed (dry)	½ cup	7
Cream cheese	1 Tbs.	16
Mozzarella, low moisture, part skim	1 oz.	18
Neufchatel	1 oz.	21
Parmesan, grated	1 oz.	27
Ricotta, part skim	1 oz.	14
Swiss	1 oz.	28

Ice Cream:

Regular, 10% fat	½ cup	27
Rich, 16% fat	½ cup	43
Ice milk	½ cup	13
Mayonnaise	1 Tbs.	10
Mayonnaise type	1 Tbs.	8
Lard	1 Tbs.	12
Frankfurter	one (2 oz.)	34

Information on the cholesterol content of foods has been taken from *Journal of the American Dietetic Association*, Vol. 61, No. 2, August 1972. (See Bibliography page 124)

GUIDELINES FOR SELECTING MARGARINE

Most margarine labels include "Nutrition Information per serving," which lists polyunsaturated and saturated fat. THE PREFERRED MARGARINES CONTAIN MORE POLYUNSATURATED THAN SATURATED FAT, in ratios greater than 1:1.

Below is nutrition information from the labels of two popular brands of margarine:

Margarine No. 1 is the preferred margarine with a ratio of 2:1

	Margarine No. 1	Margarine No. 2
Polyunsaturated Fat (in grams)	4	1
Saturated Fat (in grams)	2	2
	Ratio: 2:1	Ratio: 1:2

Soft tub and liquid margarines are likely to have better ratios than margarines in stick form. Margarines of vegetable origin CONTAIN NO CHOLESTEROL.

The guidelines above also apply to DIET OR "IMITATION" MARGARINES, which have only half the fat of regular margarines.

PART IV

LOSE WEIGHT—HELP YOUR HEALTH

About ONE THIRD OF THE POPULATION IN THE UNITED STATES IS OVERWEIGHT TO A DEGREE WHICH HAS BEEN SHOWN TO DIMINISH LIFE EXPECTANCY.

These are the facts which Dr. Beverly Winikoff of the Rockefeller Foundation reported to the U.S. Senate Select Committee on Nutrition and Human Needs.

The American Heart Association reports that obesity—if it occurs in conjunction with high blood pressure or elevated cholesterol levels—significantly increases the risk of coronary heart disease.

An important research study concluded that: Each ten percent reduction in weight in men thirty-five to fifty-five years old would result in about a twenty percent decrease in the incidence of coronary disease.

Since about 640,000 Americans die of coronary disease every year, if a decrease did occur throughout the population and were reflected in a twenty percent decrease in overall mortality, about 128,000 lives would be saved a year by reducing weight.

ENJOY LOSING WEIGHT
by Jerri Udelson, M.P.H.

Jerri Udelson, a health-care consultant who specializes in developing health programs for individuals and organizations and in assisting them to obtain funding for special projects, has contributed the following information that we feel is invaluable in helping you protect yourself against heart disease. Ms. Udelson holds a Master of Public Health degree in Health Services Administration and Health Education from Yale University.

Losing weight and keeping it off does not have to mean diets, willpower, and deprivation. Losing weight can be an opportunity for you to learn more about yourself, to change your eating habits, and to experience eating as a pleasurable activity.

People become overweight because they consume more calories than they burn up in the normal course of daily activities. A calorie is a unit of energy. *Calories that are not burned up are stored in the body in the form of fat—a pound of fat for each 3,500 excess calories.*

In order to lose one pound of fat, you must either decrease the number of calories you consume by 3,500 or else burn up 3,500 additional calories by increasing your activity level. If you cut the number of calories you consume in a day by 500, you will lose one pound in one week (7 times 500 equals 3,500). If you cut 1,000 calories from your daily diet, you will lose two pounds in one week.

Regular exercise will help you burn calories. (See Calorie-Activity Chart on pages 51 and 52.) The color-coded chart clearly shows that it is easier to lose weight by reducing calories than by exercising. Moderate exercise will help you to tone your body, to increase your circulation, and to feel healthier. Naturally, you should check with your doctor before beginning a regular exercise program.

Any weight-reduction program you choose must follow the principles of good nutrition. The basic four food groups should be included: Fruits and vegetables, meats (including fish, poultry, and eggs), cereals, and dairy products. The program should take into account your special health problems and dietary requirements, such as low saturated fat/cholesterol. And most importantly, it should take into account your food likes and dislikes and your life-style.

Anyone who wants to lose weight should be aware of how many calories he or she needs in order to maintain good health. The National Academy of Sciences has published the RECOMMENDED DIETARY ALLOWANCES (see page 91) for information on suggested number of calories in relation to height and weight.

ANALYZE YOUR EATING HABITS before beginning a weight-loss program. To do this, KEEP A FOOD DIARY FOR ONE WEEK. Write down everything you put into your mouth (including foods you eat while preparing meals or nibbles from the refrigerator). Write down the time of day, what you ate, where you were, who you were with, and how you felt when you ate (hungry, tired, bored, anxious, etc.). After several days analyze the diary. A pattern should be apparent. What circumstances trigger your eating? Are you usually hungry in the afternoon? Does the taste of one cookie lead you to an eating binge? Do you tend to eat when you are bored? Do you overeat when you are alone?

You will probably be surprised at the number of times you eat in addition to mealtimes, and at the amount of food you eat without really being hungry.

Once you have learned about your eating habits you can build a weight-loss program around them. There is no need, for example, to follow a three-meal-a-day diet, if you always skip breakfast and eat snacks in the afternoon and evening. Instead, choose low-calorie foods to snack on. *One of the easiest ways to lose weight is to reduce portions at mealtime.* Some people have lost weight by cutting normal portions in half. Then they do not feel deprived of foods they like. If you really don't like grapefruit, don't include it on your program.

LEARN TO AVOID THE CIRCUMSTANCES THAT TRIGGER YOUR EATING. If your food diary shows that you tend to eat when bored, substitute pleasurable activities for eating. These could include telephoning a friend, working on a hobby, reading a book, taking a walk, or even taking a bubble bath. If you always stop for ice cream when shopping, go for coffee instead. Don't shop for food when you are hungry. There are many ways to change your eating behavior. Some are:

● *Restrict your eating to one place in your home* and eat sitting down at the table. You will break the habit of eating while watching television, driving your car, talking on the telephone, or working at your desk.

● *Eat everything from a small plate.* This will make a portion seem bigger. Always leave something on the plate. Prove to yourself you can control your eating.

● *Eat slowly.* Chew the food and *really* taste it. Put the fork and knife down between bites.

● *Banish high-calorie foods from your house.* If you can't do this because of other family members, have your family hide them so they won't tempt you.

● *Allow yourself an occasional treat.* If you love pasta or sweets, don't deprive yourself completely. Eat small amounts of your favorite food. Savor it, and be proud of yourself for controlling your appetite.

REALLY ENJOY EATING. The next step is for

you to *experience eating as a pleasurable activity.* This exercise will help you to begin this process. Do it on a day (a weekend day, for example) when you can free yourself from normal routines.

Don't eat breakfast as soon as you wake up. Instead, wait one or more hours until you feel hunger pains in your stomach. Then get an orange and sit down by yourself at the table. Peel the orange; while you are peeling it, examine it closely. Observe its color. Feel the texture of its skin. Smell its aroma. Really involve your senses in exploring the orange rind. Examine the white membranes. When it is peeled, put it on a plate. With a knife and fork cut the orange into slices and taste a slice. Let your tongue and taste buds really *experience* the sensation of the orange. Take another slice. Close your eyes and really enjoy the taste. You've probably never tasted food this way before.

Recall this exercise frequently when you eat. You will begin to notice that you enjoy your food more, and need to eat less of it to feel satisfied.

When you plan your meals, include the basic four food groups to ensure a well-rounded diet—adequate in all essential nutrients.

Using all of these ideas you will be able to cut calories, to change the habits which work against your losing weight, and to learn to experience and to appreciate the taste of food.

Finally, embark on a weight program which is realistic. A ONE- TO TWO-POUND WEIGHT LOSS EACH WEEK is reasonable and will enable you to develop new eating patterns without going on starvation or fad diets which are impossible to follow for more than a few weeks.

If you do overeat, don't be discouraged. Take a look at what happened, and think about how you can prevent it from happening again. *Concentrate on the image of the new you.* Visualize how you will look and feel, what new clothes you will wear when you are thin, and bring this image to mind at least twice a day. If you are tempted to stray from your weight program, see if you can conjure up this picture and it will reinforce your determination to succeed. Reward yourself as you progress. Treat yourself to a piece of clothing, perfume, a new book, or something you want. Congratulate yourself on your success.

HOW LONG WILL IT TAKE
TO "BURN UP" CALORIES

Check the chart below to determine HOW MANY MINUTES it will take for you to "burn up" the calories in each food.

CALORIE-ACTIVITY CHART

FOOD AND CALORIES	ACTIVITY*			
	Walking	Bicycling	Swimming	Running
Apple (one, medium) 61 calories	12	7	5	3
Apple pie (⅙ of pie) 231 calories	44	28	21	11
Fresh halibut (broiled) 4 oz. 114 calories	22	14	10	6
"Fast foods" fish sandwich 400 calories	77	49	36	21
Fresh broccoli (½ cup) with lemon juice (1 Tbs.) 24 calories	5	3	2	1
Frozen broccoli (½ cup) with Hollandaise sauce 121 calories	23	15	11	6
Broiled chicken (4 oz.) 188 calories	36	23	17	10
Frozen chicken pot pie (8 oz.) 450 calories	86½	55	40	23

*Energy cost for 150-pound individual.

CALORIE-ACTIVITY CHART
FOOD AND CALORIES   ACTIVITY*

Food and Calories	Walking	Bicycling	Swimming	Running
Skim milk (8 oz.) 86 calories	16½	10	8	4
Whole milk, 3.7% (8 oz.) 157 calories	30	13	14	8
Lean smoked ham (4 oz.) 212 calories	41	26	19	11
Pork spareribs (4 oz.) 499 calories	96	61	44½	26
Angel food cake (1/12th of whole) 137 calories	26	17	12	7
White cake (1/12th of whole) 333 calories	64	41	30	17
1% low-fat cottage cheese 82 calories	16	10	7	4
Creamed cottage cheese 117 calories	22½	14	10	6

Energy cost of activities per minute:	Walking	5.2 calories
	Bicycling	8.2 calories
	Swimming	11.2 calories
	Running	19.4 calories

PART V

LOW-FAT/LOW-CALORIE COOKING GUIDE

COOKING TIPS

Learn to cook with wines and herbs instead of butter. Use the Flavor-Magic chart on pages 54 and 55 for new ways to flavor foods.

Broil, bake, or poach fish instead of frying.

Buy tuna fish packed in water instead of oil.

Substitute low-fat yogurt and low-fat milk for cream and regular milk in recipes.

Buy canned fruits in unsweetened juice instead of heavy syrup, cutting down on sugar intake and calories.

WHEN COOKING MEATS:

First, trim off all fat. Broil or roast meat. Use a rack to drain off fat.

When meat needs to be browned first, try browning under the broiler instead of in a pan.

Use a Teflon pan to fry meats, to eliminate extra calories.

Stews, meat casseroles, and soups should be cooked a day ahead. After food has been refrigerated, remove hardened fat from the top. If in a hurry, use ice cubes to congeal the fat.

Serve meats without gravies or sauces.

Cut off fat and remove skin from poultry before cooking.

Try the low-fat recipes beginning on page 57.

FLAVOR-MAGIC CHART

Match each flavor with the food listed below: Read across each row to find "Flavor Magic" for each food.

Green-Light Flavors	Lemon Juice	Red Wine	White Wine	Sherry Wine	Garlic Fresh/ Powder	Chives/ Onion Powder
Beef		●		●	●	●
Chicken	●	●	●	●	●	●
Lamb		●			●	●
Pork			●	●		●
Veal	●		●	●	●	●
Fish, Shellfish	●		●		●	●
Salad Dressings	●	●	●		●	●
Vegetables:						
Asparagus	●		●			●
Beets						
Broccoli	●				●	●
Carrots	●			●		
Eggplant					●	●
Green Beans	●				●	●
Lima Beans						●
Mushrooms	●	●	●		●	●
Potatoes						●
Spinach	●				●	●
Squash				●		
Sweet Potatoes				●		
Tomatoes		●	●		●	●
Zucchini		●			●	●

Jams Jellies	Bay Leaf	Basil	Dill	Ginger	Thyme	Dry Mustard
Apricot	●	●	●		●	●
			●	●	●	●
Pineapple	●	●	●	●		
Plum		●	●	●		●
Currant		●	●		●	
	●	●	●	●	●	●
	●	●	●			●
Orange		●				●
		●	●	●	●	●
		●				●
Currant	●	●	●	●	●	
	●	●	●			
	●	●	●		●	
	●					●
	●	●	●			●
		●	●			●
	●	●				
Pineapple			●	●		
Orange/ Apricot				●		
	●	●	●		●	●
	●	●	●			

TRIM MEATS TO
SAVE CALORIES

The chart below shows how you can drastically cut your calories by trimming fats from meats. The column on the far right lists the *number of calories you can save per serving.*

MEATS (from legs)	TOTAL CALORIES OF 4 OZ. COOKED SERVING		CALORIES SAVED BY TRIMMING FAT
	UNTRIMMED	TRIMMED	
VEAL	267	245	22
LAMB	317	211	106
RUMP OF BEEF	394	236	158
FRESH HAM (PORK)	424	246	178
BEEF: Round	296	214	182
Chuck (arm and round bone)	328	219	109
Sirloin	439	235	204
T-Bone	537	253	284
Porterhouse	527	254	273
Rib Roast	499	273	226

GREEN-LIGHT RECIPES
LOW IN SATURATED FAT/CHOLESTEROL

The recipes on the following pages demonstrate that you can cut down on saturated fat/cholesterol and calories in foods without any loss of flavor.

These main dish recipes *DO NOT INCLUDE SALT* as an ingredient because many people need to watch their salt intake. For additional low-salt recipes see the LOW-SALT-LIVING GUIDE by the same authors.

The calorie contents of the recipes were calculated by the HVH-CWRU Nutrient Data Base of Case Western Reserve University in Cleveland, Ohio.

The calorie values on these recipes are based on the use of precise and accurate measurements. However, when an ingredient is termed "medium" or "large" in a recipe, it means that the Nutrient Data Base has given it an approximate value. The size of a "medium" ingredient you use at home may differ from the one analyzed by the Data Base, so calorie values may vary slightly.

BEEF BURGUNDY
(4 servings)

1   pound lean round steak
       (cut into 1-inch cubes)
1   Tbs. flour
1   Tbs. vegetable oil
1   onion (diced)
1   bay leaf
6   peppercorns

        ¼ tsp. thyme
        ¼ tsp. marjoram
        ¾ cup red wine
        ¼ cup water
        1 cup fresh mushrooms (sliced)
        1 tsp. parsley flakes

Sprinkle flour over meat. Brown meat and onion in hot oil. When browned, add bay leaf, peppercorns, thyme, marjoram, wine, and water. Cover pan and cook over medium heat for 1 hour, or until meat is tender. Then add mushrooms and parsley. Continue cooking covered, for 10 minutes more.

One 4 oz. serving of Beef Burgundy contains 217 calories.

VEAL WITH HERBS   (4 servings)

        1 pound veal steak or cutlet
        2 Tbs. vegetable oil
        2 medium onions (sliced)
        1 clove garlic (crushed)
        3 Tbs. water
        3 Tbs. lemon juice
        1 tsp. oregano
        1 Tbs. parsley flakes
        1 Tbs. paprika

Place oil in pan. Brown meat on both sides. Add remaining ingredients. Cover pan and simmer slowly for 30 minutes, or until meat is tender. Serve with lemon slices and chopped parsley.

One 4 oz. serving of Veal With Herbs contains 263 calories.

SHERRIED VEAL
(4 servings)

1 pound veal for scallopini
   (thin sliced)
½ tsp. pepper
2 Tbs. flour
2 Tbs. vegetable oil
½ pound fresh mushrooms (sliced)
1 clove garlic (crushed)
1 Tbs. lemon juice
4 Tbs. sherry wine

Sprinkle pepper and flour over meat. Heat oil in pan and brown meat until golden brown. Add mushrooms, garlic, and lemon juice. Cover pan and cook over medium heat for 10 minutes. Add wine and cook, covered, an additional 10 minutes.

One 4 oz. serving of Sherried Veal contains 286 calories.

LAMB WITH APPLES AND CURRY (4 servings)

1 pound shoulder of lamb (boneless)
   (cut into 1-inch cubes)
1 Tbs. vegetable oil
1 large onion (chopped)
1 cup water
½ tsp. pepper
½ tsp. oregano
½ tsp. cinnamon
½ tsp. curry powder
2 Tbs. lemon juice
2 apples, peeled, cored, and quartered
dash of parsley and paprika

Place oil in pan. Brown meat and onions in hot oil. When browned, add water, pepper, oregano, cinnamon, curry, and lemon juice. Cover pan and cook over medium heat for 40 minutes, or until meat is tender. Then add apples and simmer another 10 minutes. Garnish with parsley and paprika.

One 4 oz. serving of Lamb With Apples and Curry is 207 calories.

LOW-CAL KEBABS

Skewer meat, chicken, or fish. Mix and match with your favorite vegetable, fruit, and herbs.

Calories (Cal.) are given per serving.

Use suggested herbs from Flavor-Magic Chart to add to marinades (see pages 54 and 55).

Marinade for Lamb and Beef (4 servings)	Marinade for Chicken (4 servings)
½ cup red wine	½ cup plain yogurt
¼ cup vegetable oil	3 Tbs. lemon juice
1 clove garlic, crushed	1 clove garlic, crushed

Marinate meats or chicken overnight in refrigerator. Next day drain marinade; alternate meat or poultry on skewer with vegetables or fruits. Broil over charcoal or in oven.

Marinade for Fish	FISH: (4 oz. serving)
½ cup white wine	Scallops — 92 Cal.
¼ cup vegetable oil	Haddock — 90 Cal.
½ tsp. pepper	Halibut — 114 Cal.
½ tsp. dill weed	Snapper — 106 Cal.
½ tsp. tarragon	(Cut into 2″ cubes with skin on)

Place fish in marinade and refrigerate for 1-2 hours. Drain marinade; alternate fish on skewer with vegetables or fruits. Broil over charcoal or in oven.

Eggplant Cubes — ½ cup — 19 Cal.
Green Pepper (one-half) — 9 Cal.
Mushrooms — ½ cup — 10 Cal.
Onion — ¼ cup — 16 Cal.
Pineapple Chunks (in own juice) — ¼ cup — 24 Cal.
Potato (partially boiled) — ½ cup — 59 Cal.
Tomato — (one medium) — 27 Cal.

CHICKEN HAWAIIAN
(4 servings)

Two 8 oz. chicken breasts
    (cut into halves)
1 cup crushed pineapple
    in its own juice
½ cup orange marmalade
¼ teaspoon ginger
1 clove garlic (crushed)
dash of nutmeg

Remove skin from chicken. Place chicken in baking pan. Cover chicken with pineapple, pineapple juice, and marmalade. Add garlic and ginger, sprinkle nutmeg on top. Cook, uncovered, in 350-degree oven for 30 minutes, or until chicken is tender. Baste occasionally with sauce from pineapple and marmalade.

One 4 oz. serving of Chicken Hawaiian contains 328 calories.

CHICKEN IN RED WINE
(4 servings)

Two 8 oz. chicken breasts
   (cut into halves)
½ tsp. pepper
4 Tbs. flour
2 Tbs. margarine
2 cloves garlic (crushed)
1 cup red wine
4 small onions (quartered)
½ pound whole fresh mushrooms

Remove skin from chicken. Season chicken with pepper and dredge in flour. Heat margarine in pan and brown chicken on both sides; remove to casserole. Add garlic, wine, onions, and mushrooms to drippings in the pan. Bring to a boil; then pour over chicken. Bake covered in 350-degree oven for 30 minutes. Baste occasionally. Remove cover and bake uncovered another 10 minutes.

One 4 oz. serving of Chicken in Red Wine contains 359 calories.

FRESH FISH FILLETS IN FOIL
(4 servings)

4   fish fillets (4 oz. each)
1½ tsp. margarine
½   cup mushrooms (sliced)
¼   cup green onions (sliced)
1   Tbs. parsley flakes
1   tsp. paprika
½   cup dry white wine
2   Tbs. lemon juice

Preheat oven to 400 degrees. Cut heavy aluminum foil into rectangular piece 18" × 12" and fold up edges to make a baking pan. Lightly grease inside of foil and place fish fillets (skin side down) on top of greased foil. Cover fish with mushrooms, onions, and parsley. Sprinkle paprika on top. Pour over wine and lemon juice. Draw edges of foil together and seal. Bake in oven for 20 minutes, or until fish flakes easily with a fork. Serve fish in foil.

One 4 oz. serving of Fish Fillets in Foil contains 128 calories.

PART VI

COLOR-CODED DINING-OUT GUIDE

ON LOW-SATURATED-FAT/ LOW-CHOLESTEROL FOODS

Some people on diets low in saturated fat/cholesterol think that they cannot go to a restaurant because there will be few foods on the menu that they are allowed.

Although there are some foods that must be avoided either at home or when eating out, there is still a wide variety of foods that can be selected from the menu of your favorite restaurant.

This section on dining out gives you an easy color-coded guide to choosing foods in restaurants. *The foods listed in* GREEN *are low in saturated fat/cholesterol content and may be eaten often; those in* YELLOW *are moderate and may be eaten as an occasional treat; and those in* RED *are high and should be avoided.*

Read the color-coded selections for breakfast, lunch, and dinner on the following pages, and make your selections from those foods listed in GREEN.

Don't miss the specialty-restaurant menus: Italian, French, Greek, and Delicatessen; and the exclusive Fast-Foods section.

AIRLINE TRAVEL THE LOW-FAT WAY

Most airlines have meals available for passengers upon request that are low fat/cholesterol. Be sure to order your special meal when you make your ticket reservation. Some airlines require 24 hours advance notice.

BREAKFAST, LUNCH, AND DINNER MENUS

If your doctor has recommended a special diet, use this guide to consult with your doctor or dietitian before dining out.

BREAKFAST

All fruits and fruit juices	
Most ready-to-eat cereals with skim milk	"Natural" cereals Cereals with whole milk
Smoked ham (lean)	Bacon, sausage
Waffles with syrup Pancakes with syrup Smoked salmon	French toast Eggs—a concentrated source of cholesterol
Toast with margarine English muffin Bagel Melba toast Jelly, marmalade, honey	Toast with butter Croissant Doughnut Danish pastry Cream cheese
Nondairy creamer Margarine	Cream Butter
Coffee, tea, skim milk, buttermilk	Whole milk

Eat moderate amounts of:

Canadian bacon

SOUPS: Vegetable, beef, chicken	Cream soups
SANDWICHES: Lean roast beef Lean pastrami Lean tongue Chicken (sliced) Chicken salad Turkey (sliced) Turkey salad Tunafish salad Salmon salad Crab salad Baked ham Smoked salmon	**SANDWICHES:** Hamburger Cheeseburger Corned beef Deviled ham Egg salad Frankfurter Chopped liver Bacon Fried fish Cream cheese Grilled cheese
FISH: Broiled or baked with mar- garine Baked potato with margarine	**FISH:** Fried or broiled with butter Baked potato with butter
Julienne salad (without egg yolk or cheese) Fruit salad with sherbet Cole slaw Chili con carne Spaghetti with tomato sauce	Julienne salad with egg yolk and cheese Cheese dishes: quiche, souffle, Welsh rabbit Potato chips Potato salad Pizza
Low-fat cottage cheese (1–2% fat) Coffee, tea, skim milk Buttermilk Fruit juices Soft drinks	Spaghetti with meatballs Creamed cottage cheese (6% fat) Milkshakes Whole milk

Eat moderate amounts of: Shrimp, olives, avocado, sardines, bologna, cottage cheese (4% or less fat), french fried potatoes

DINNER

Appetizers

Fresh or canned fruit	
Fruit juices	
Oysters, clams, crab	Chopped liver
Pickled herring	Paté (Goose liver)
Smoked salmon, lobster	
SOUPS: Vegetable, beef, chicken	SOUPS: Cream soups

Main Course

Beef tenderloin, filet mignon, lean sirloin	Standing rib roast, rib steak, club steak
	Beef or calves' liver
Veal with wine	Veal with cheese
Veal with mushrooms	Veal breast
	Sweetbreads
Lean ham	Spareribs, pork chops
Turkey (roasted)	Turkey with cream or cheese sauce
Chicken (roasted or broiled). Remove skin before eating.	Chicken, fried, or with cream or cheese sauce

Lamb chops or leg of lamb	Lamb breast
FISH: Broiled or baked with lemon, margarine	FISH: Fried, broiled with butter or baked with butter
SHELLFISH: Crab, lobster, scallops, broiled or poached in wine	SHELLFISH: Scallops, fried or in cream sauce
Fruit or lettuce salad	Salad accompaniments: Shredded or crumbled cheese
Salad dressings	

Vegetables

Baked potato with margarine	Scalloped and creamed potatoes
Hashbrown potatoes	
Fresh, frozen or canned vegetables with margarine	Vegetables with butter, cream, or cheese sauce

Eat moderate amounts of:

Shrimp (plain, boiled)	Canadian bacon

DESSERTS

Fresh fruit	Ice cream, sundaes, pies, pastries, cakes, tortes, whipped cream, crème caramel, mousse
Sherbet, gelatin	
Nondairy pressurized topping	
Angel food cake (unfrosted)	

SPECIALTY RESTAURANTS
ITALIAN

Appetizers

Minestrone soup
Fish soup with
tomatoes
Melon and Pro-
sciutto
Boiled ham
Coponata (diced
eggplant)

Antipasto (with
cheese and
sausage)
Cheese-stuffed
mushrooms
Cheese-stuffed
clams
Chicken livers

Main Course

PASTAS:
Spaghetti,
Linguini:
Tomato sauce
Meat sauce
Clam sauce (red
or white)
Anchovy sauce
Ravioli with meat
Chicken caccia-
tore
Chicken in wine
Veal with mush-
rooms
Veal with lemon
Veal with wine
Filet of beef with
wine
Stuffed eggplant
Roasted Italian
peppers

PASTAS:
Fettucini (with
cream, butter,
cheese)
Lasagna
Canneloni and
manicotti with
cheese
Spaghetti with
butter
Spaghetti with
sausage
Veal parmesan
(cheese)

Baked eggplant
Parmigiana
Stuffed peppers
with meat and
cheese

Desserts

Sherbet

Biscuit tortoni,
zabaglione

FRENCH

Appetizers

Bouillabaisse
  (fish soup)
Consommé
Crudités (raw
  vegetables)
Oysters, clams,
  scallops in wine

Seafood bisque
French onion soup

Escargots (butter
  sauce)
Paté (goose, pork
  liver)

Main Course

Filet of beef
  (tournedos)
Rack of lamb
  (chops)
Scallops of veal

MEAT SAUCES:
  Madeira (wine
    and mush-
    rooms)
  Diable
    (mustard)
  Wine: Bour-
    guignon
Chicken with red
  wine (Coq au
  vin)

Lobster, broiled,
  or boiled
All fish: baked,
  poached, or
  broiled

MEATS SERVED
  WITH SAUCES:
  Béarnaise
    (eggs, butter)
  Bêchamel (but-
    ter, milk)
  Bordelaise (salt
    pork)
  Mornay
    (cheese)
  Rémoulade
    (egg yolks)

Chicken with
  cheese or
  cream sauce
Duck
Sweetbreads
Veal with cheese
Stuffed pork
Seafood: Thermi-
  dor, crêpes,
  quiches
Fish with cheese
  or butter sauce

GREEK

Avgolemono (lemon-flavored soup)

Greek salad
Cucumbers with low-fat yogurt

Rice stuffed grape leaves
Gyro sandwich
Shashlik
Shish-ke-bob

Greek Easter soup

Spinach-cheese pastry
Moussaka (eggplant with cheese, eggs)
Baked eggplant with meats and cheese

Baklava, cheese pastry

DELICATESSEN*

Chicken noodle soup
Mushroom-barley soup
Cabbage soup

Pickled herring

Smoked salmon
Smoked whitefish
Lean pastrami
Lean tongue

Turkey
Chicken
Cole slaw
Health slaw salad
Pickles
Sauerkraut

Chicken soup with matzo balls
Borsht with sour cream

Herring in sour cream

Salami
Corned beef
Liverwurst
Chopped chicken liver
Potato salad
Sliced cheese
Cheese blintzes
Potato pancakes

*Many delicatessen foods are very high in sodium content.

FAST-FOOD RESTAURANTS

Responding to consumer requests for nutrition information, the following restaurant chains have completed nutrient analyses and made them available as a public service. Data from other fast-food chains were not completed at the time of publication, and cannot be included.

The calories, fat content, and cholesterol are given in servings. The serving size (weight) is in grams, and fat content is in grams (g.). The cholesterol is in milligrams (mgs.).

McDONALD'S*

ITEM	SERVING WEIGHT (g.)	CALORIES	CHOLESTEROL (mgs.)	FAT (g.)
Hamburger	99.3	260	25	10
Cheeseburger	114.2	300	40	13
Quarter-Pounder	163.8	420	70	21
Quarter-Pounder with cheese	193.4	520	95	29
Big Mac	186.7	540	75	31
Filet-O-Fish	131.3	400	45	23
French Fries	69.3	210	10	11
Hashbrown Potatoes	58.1	130	10	8
Chocolate Shake	288.9	360	30	9

*Reproduced with permission of McDonald's Corporation 1977, 1978.

FAST-FOOD RESTAURANTS
(continued)

ITEM	SERVING WEIGHT (g.)	CALORIES	CHOLESTEROL (mgs.)	FAT (g.)
Vanilla Shake	288.7	320	30	8
Strawberry Shake	292.6	340	30	8
Apple Pie	91.4	300	15	19
Cherry Pie	92.4	300	15	18
McDonald-Land Cookies	63.4	290	10	11
Hot Fudge Sundae	151.2	290	20	10
Caramel Sundae	144.6	280	20	7
Strawberry Sundae	144.2	230	20	4
Pineapple Sundae	144.1	230	20	5
Egg McMuffin	132.4	350	190	20
Hot Cakes with Butter/Syrup	205.9	470	35	9
Scrambled Eggs	77.3	160	300	12
Pork Sausage	48.1	180	45	17
English Muffin (buttered)	61.9	190	10	6

DAIRY QUEEN*

ITEM	SERVING WEIGHT (g.)	CALORIES	CHOLESTEROL (mgs.)	FAT (g.)
Big Brazier Deluxe	213	470	—	24
Big Brazier Regular	184	457	—	23
Big Brazier/cheese	213	553	—	30
Brazier with cheese	121	318	—	14
Chili Dog	128	330	—	20
Brazier Dog	99	273	—	15
Brazier Regular	106	260	—	9
Super Brazier	298	783	—	48
Super Brazier Dog	182	518	—	30
Super Brazier Dog with cheese	203	593	—	36
Super Brazier Chili Dog	210	555	—	33

---

*1978 Data. No data available on cholesterol content.

FAST-FOOD RESTAURANTS
(continued)

The calories, fat content, and cholesterol are given in servings. The serving size is per unit, and the fat content is in grams (g). The cholesterol is in milligrams (mgs.).

PIZZA HUT*
THIN'N CRISPY PIZZA (2 slices from 13″ pie)

A SERVING

ITEM	SERVING	CALORIES	CHOLESTEROL (mgs.)	FAT (g.)
Standard Cheese	one	340	—	10
SuperStyle Cheese	one	410	—	14
Standard Pepperoni	one	370	—	16
SuperStyle Pepperoni	one	430	—	19
Standard Pork with Mushrooms	one	380	—	14
SuperStyle Pork with Mushrooms	one	450	—	19
Supreme	one	400	—	16
Super Supreme	one	510	—	25

---

*1979 data.

WENDY'S*

ITEM	SERVING WEIGHT (g.)	CALORIES	CHOLESTEROL (mgs.)	FAT (g.)
Hamburger (single)	200	472	69	26
Hamburger (double)	285	669	124	40
Hamburger (triple)	360	853	207	51
Single Cheese	240	577	88	34
Double Cheese	325	797	156	48
Triple Cheese	400	1036	224	68
Chili	250	229	26	8
French Fries	120	327	6	16
Frosty	250	391	45	16

*1979 data.

FAST-FOOD RESTAURANTS
(continued)

ARBY'S*

ITEM	SERVING WEIGHT	CALORIES	CHOLESTEROL (mgs.)	FAT (g.)
Roast Beef	5 oz.	350	30	15
Beef & Cheese	6 oz.	450	35	22
Super Roast Beef	9.75 oz.	620	30	28
Swiss King	9.25 oz.	660	40	34
Ham 'N Cheese	5.50 oz.	380	40	17
Turkey	6 oz.	410	40	19
Turkey Deluxe	8.51 oz.	510	30	24
Club	9 oz.	560	40	30

KENTUCKY FRIED CHICKEN**

3-Piece Dinner: Chicken (3 pieces), Mashed Potatoes and Gravy, Cole Slaw, and Roll.

Original Recipe	15.0 oz.	830	285	46
Extra Crispy	15.4 oz.	950	265	54

*1979 data.
**1976 data.

The calories, fat content, and cholesterol are given in servings. The serving size is per unit, and the fat content is in grams (g). The cholesterol is in milligrams (mgs.)

BURGER KING*

ITEM	SERVING	CALORIES	CHOLESTEROL (mgs.)	FAT (g.)
Hamburger	one	290	—	13
Cheeseburger	one	350	—	17
Double Cheeseburger	one	530	—	31
**Whopper Jr.	one	370	—	20
**Whopper Jr. with cheese	one	420	—	25
**Whopper	one	630	—	36
**Whopper/cheese	one	740	—	45
Double Beef Whopper	one	850	—	52
Double Beef Whopper with cheese	one	950	—	60
French Fries	one	210	—	11
Onion Rings	one	270	—	16
Apple pie	one	240	—	12
Chocolate shake	one	340	—	10
Vanilla shake	one	340	—	11

*1979 data. No data available on cholesterol content.
**To reduce calories sandwiches may be ordered without mayonnaise.

PART VII

THE DOCTOR ANSWERS QUESTIONS ON DIET AND HEART DISEASE

by Abby G. Abelson, M.D.

Americans are becoming increasingly aware of the effect of saturated fat/cholesterol on their health, and are seeking information from their doctors concerning their diet and their health. Some of the most frequently asked questions are answered on the following pages by Abby G. Abelson, M.D.

CONSULT YOUR OWN PHYSICIAN FOR DIET RECOMMENDATIONS FOR YOUR INDIVIDUAL HEALTH NEEDS.

Q. WHAT IS FAT?

A. Fat is a substance found in many plant and animal foods. Fat is a concentrated energy source for our bodies. The body can store the fats we eat if the energy is not needed immediately.

Q. WHAT DOES FAT DO IN THE BODY?

A. In addition to being a storehouse for energy, fat is needed for many body functions. Fat is essential in the formation of hormones, chemicals that regulate the processes of growth, sexual maturity, and pregnancy. Fat also helps carry some vitamins (A,D,E,and K) through the blood. Fat serves as insulation, helping the body to conserve heat. It also functions as padding, protecting the body from injury.

Q. SHOULD I HAVE SOME FAT IN MY DIET?

A. Yes. Fat is a concentrated energy source providing nine calories per gram, more than twice the energy provided by carbohydrates or protein.

Q. HOW MUCH FAT SHOULD I BE EATING?

A. Most Americans eat too much fat. The Senate Select Committee on Nutrition and Human Needs recommends in its *Dietary Goals* that Americans should reduce the amount of total fat—from the forty percent of total calories now consumed to only thirty percent of calorie intake.

Q. IS THERE MORE THAN ONE TYPE OF FAT IN FOODS?

A. Yes. There are saturated fats, polyunsaturated fats, and cholesterol.

Q. WHAT FOODS CONTAIN SATURATED FAT?

A. Saturated fat is found mainly in foods from animal sources, such as meats and dairy products. It is also found in a few vegetable sources, such as coconut oil, palm oil, and cocoa butter.

Q. WHAT ARE POLYUNSATURATED FATS?

A. Polyunsaturated fats are from vegetable sources. They are usually oils (liquid at room temperature) such as safflower, sunflower, sesame, corn, soybean, peanut, and cottonseed.

Q. WHAT IS CHOLESTEROL?

A. Cholesterol is a fatty substance that is made only in animal tissues. We get most of it into our bodies by eating animal foods, such as meats and dairy products. Cholesterol is found *ONLY* in foods from animal sources. Foods from plant sources do not contain cholesterol.

Q. WHERE ELSE DOES CHOLESTEROL COME FROM?

A. Your liver can make cholesterol. In fact, after the age of six months, your liver can manufacture enough cholesterol to meet your body's needs. Some cholesterol is also manufactured by the intestine.

Q. WHAT DOES CHOLESTEROL DO IN THE BODY?

A. Cholesterol is one form in which fats circulate in your blood. It has many functions. Cholesterol comprises much of the material in your brain and nervous system. The body uses it to manufacture many hormones, including the sex hormones.

Q. HOW DO FATS TRAVEL THROUGH THE BODY?

A. Fats must be attached to proteins to be transported through the blood to the body areas where they are needed.

Q. WHAT IS SERUM CHOLESTEROL?

A. Serum cholesterol is the cholesterol carried in the liquid portion of the blood.

Q. HOW DO I KNOW WHAT MY SERUM CHO-
LESTEROL LEVEL IS?

A. Serum cholesterol level is measured from a
blood sample through a chemical test ordered
by your physician who will inform you if your
cholesterol level is in the normal range.

Q. IS THERE CAUSE FOR CONCERN IF MY
CHOLESTEROL LEVEL IS HIGH?

A. Many studies show that people with high levels
of serum cholesterol have an increased risk of
coronary heart disease, heart attacks, and stroke.

Q. WHAT IS CORONARY HEART DISEASE?

A. Coronary heart disease is a disease of the coronary arteries. It means that the coronary arteries are involved with atherosclerosis.

Q. WHAT ARE THE CORONARY ARTERIES?

A. The coronary arteries are the tubes or blood
vessels that carry blood to the heart muscle.

Q. WHAT IS ATHEROSCLEROSIS?

A. Atherosclerosis is the process that many people refer to as "hardening of the arteries." It
is a buildup of fatty materials along the inner
walls of the arteries to the heart. This buildup
is like the deposits of minerals on the inside
of a water pipe. It is a very slow process that
may go on for many years without causing
symptoms.

Q. WHY IS ATHEROSCLEROSIS A HEALTH
PROBLEM?

A. The buildup of fatty materials on the artery walls gradually narrows the arteries. As a result there is a decrease of blood flow to the body's organs. When the blood flow from the coronary artery to an area of the heart muscle is blocked, the result is a heart attack. When the artery flow leading to the brain is blocked, the result is a stroke.

Q. WHAT IS A HEART ATTACK?

A. A heart attack (called a "myocardial infarction" by physicians) happens when blood flow through a coronary artery stops. The stoppage is usually caused by a blood clot in an area of atherosclerosis.

The blockage of blood flow results in the death of cells in the heart muscle previously supplied by the artery. This area of cells dies because it can no longer get blood or oxygen.

Q. WHAT HAPPENS AFTER A HEART ATTACK?

A. What happens after a heart attack varies with the size of the area of heart muscle affected. The area affected may not pump the blood with as much force as before. If blood supply is interrupted to the cells that are involved in making the heart beat, an irregular heartbeat can result.

Q. CAN THE HEART HEAL AFTER A HEART ATTACK?

A. After a heart attack, scar tissue forms over the injured area, the same way a cut on your arm heals.

Q. WHAT ELSE CAN RESULT FROM NARROWED CORONARY ARTERIES?

A. Narrowed (but unclogged) coronary arteries may not be able to carry enough oxygen to the heart muscle at times of hard work or emotional upset. This temporary lack of oxygen may cause heart pain (angina) or a disturbance in the rhythm of the heart.

Q. WHAT FACTORS CONTRIBUTE TO AN INCREASED RISK OF HEART ATTACK AND STROKE?

A. The American Heart Association identifies several "risk factors" that contribute to an increased risk of heart attack and stroke. Some of these risk factors cannot be changed:

> HEREDITY—"A tendency toward these problems can be inherited."
>
> SEX—Men are more susceptible than women before the menopause. After menopause, heart attack rates for women increase sharply, but never reach that of men.
>
> AGE—The death rates go up with age.
>
> RACE—Black Americans are twice as likely to have high blood pressure as whites. High blood pressure contributes to heart attack and stroke, and blacks suffer more strokes at an earlier age and with more severe results.

Q. ARE THERE ANY RISK FACTORS WHICH I CAN CONTROL?

A. Yes. Although some risk factors are beyond your control, you can change others (with medical supervision):

High serum cholesterol may be lowered with a diet low in saturated fat/cholesterol.

High blood pressure may be controlled with diet and medication.

The important thing to remember is that the *DANGER OF HEART ATTACK AND STROKE INCREASES WITH THE NUMBER OF RISK FACTORS PRESENT.*

So it makes good sense to do away with any risk factor that you have the power to change.

One of the easiest risk factors to change is your diet.

Q. WHAT CHANGE IN MY DIET IS RECOMMENDED?

A. The American Heart Association states:

A balanced diet low in saturated fat and cholesterol, which contains the number of calories needed to maintain optimal body weight, will help reduce the risk of heart attack and stroke and prevent overweight as well.

Q. WHAT DOES SATURATED FAT HAVE TO DO WITH SERUM (BLOOD) CHOLESTEROL?

A. The level of saturated fat in the diet is of concern because it has been directly linked to high levels of blood cholesterol, and therefore to an increased risk of heart disease.

Q. CAN DIET REALLY AFFECT MY CHANCES OF GETTING A HEART ATTACK?

A. Studies from all over the world show a close correlation between the consumption of saturated fat (mostly dairy and meat fats) and the death rate from coronary heart disease.

Q. HOW DO POLYUNSATURATED FATS AFFECT BLOOD CHOLESTEROL?

A. Polyunsaturated fats in the diet lower serum cholesterol. By lowering serum cholesterol, they decrease the rate of atherosclerosis, thereby decreasing the risk of heart attack and stroke.

Q. CAN THE PROPORTION OF POLYUNSATURATES IN THE DIET AFFECT CORONARY HEART DISEASE?

A. Yes, definitely. In a twelve-year-long study in Finland, researchers found that replacement of dairy fats in the diet with vegetable oils—that is, substituting polyunsaturates for saturated fats—resulted in a substantial reduction in deaths in men from coronary heart disease.

Q. HOW MUCH OF MY DAILY FAT INTAKE SHOULD BE IN SATURATED FAT?

A. Saturated fat should only account for about ten percent of total energy intake, according to the *Dietary Goals*.

Q. HOW MUCH OF MY DAILY FAT INTAKE SHOULD BE IN POLYUNSATURATED FAT?

A. The *Dietary Goals* recommends that polyunsaturated fats should account for about ten percent of energy intake.

Q. SHOULD DIETARY CHOLESTEROL BE REDUCED?

A. The *Dietary Goals* recommends a reduction of dietary cholesterol to about 300 mgs. a day. Since the average daily diet in the United States contains about twice that amount (600 mgs. a day), they recommend reducing the amount of cholesterol in the diet by one half!

The yolk of one egg contains 250 mgs. of cholesterol—almost the total daily intake recommended by the *Dietary Goals*. Since cholesterol is present in foods from animals (which are sources of protein), careful planning is necessary to lower your cholesterol intake while continuing to maintain adequate protein intake.

Q. CAN THERE BE A HARMFUL EFFECT FROM FOLLOWING A LOW-FAT DIET?

A. No, according to the American Heart Association, which reported:

> Diets similar to those recommended (with lowered calories, saturated fat, and cholesterol) have been consumed by many persons in the United States for periods of more than fifteen years without any evidence of harmful effects. Worldwide population studies have yielded similar findings.

Q. SHOULD A DIET LOW IN SATURATED FAT/ CHOLESTEROL BE STARTED IN CHILDHOOD TO PREVENT ATHEROSCLEROSIS IN LATER LIFE?

A. The American Heart Association reports that "dietary habits formed during the developing years may continue lifelong and influence the severity of atherosclerosis in later life."

The Heart Association notes the fact that nutritional requirements differ during certain periods of growth and development. Therefore, consult your child's doctor to determine if a diet low in saturated fat/cholesterol meets your child's individual health needs.

Q. HOW CAN I MAKE THESE RECOMMENDED CHANGES IN MY DIET?

A. By changing your food shopping and eating habits you can reduce your total fat consumption; *decrease the proportion of saturated fat in the diet; increase the proportion of polyunsaturates, and decrease your cholesterol intake.*

Q. DOES MY BEING OVERWEIGHT HAVE ANY EFFECT ON MY HEART?

A. Yes, overweight (obesity) influences your heart in three basic ways:

1. It is often associated with a high blood-cholesterol level, which increases the severity of atherosclerosis.
2. It is associated with high blood pressure, which accelerates the atherosclerosis in all of the blood vessels, including the coronary arteries.
3. It adds to the heart's workload by making the heart pump more blood through a larger blood-vessel system.

DECREASING WEIGHT IF YOU ARE OVERWEIGHT MAY LOWER THIS STRAIN ON YOUR HEART.

Q. DO I HAVE TO CONSULT WITH MY DOCTOR BEFORE TAKING AN ANTACID OR DECONGESTANT OR OTHER OVER-THE-COUNTER DRUG?

A. Absolutely. It is *very important* to consult your physician before taking any over-the-counter non-prescription drug if you are taking any medication for any illness—particularly coronary heart disease or high blood pressure.

MEDICAL BIBLIOGRAPHY

American Heart Association Publications:

Coronary Risk Handbook, 1973

Diet and Coronary Heart Disease, 1978

Heart Attack, Pamphlet, 1972

Heart Facts, 1978 and 1979

Stroke Risk Handbook, 1974

Brown, Helen B., Ph.D., "Current Focus on Fat in the Diet." White Paper, American Dietetic Association, 1977.

Dietary Goals for the United States. Second Edition. Select Committee on Nutrition and Human Needs, United States Senate. U. S. Government Printing Office, Washington, D.C., December 1977.

"Fats in Foods and Diet." U.S. Dept. of Agriculture, *Information Bulletin* No. 361.

Glueck, C.J. and Conner, W.E., "Diet-Coronary Heart Disease Relationships Reconnoitered." *The American Journal of Clinical Nutrition*, 31, pp. 727–737, May 1978.

Glueck, C.J., Mattson, F., and Bierman, E.L., "Diet and Coronary Heart Disease: Another View." *New England Journal of Medicine*, 298: 26, pp. 1471–1474, 1978.

Kannel, W.B., Castelli, W.P., Gordon, T., and McNamara, P.M., "Serum Cholesterol, Lipoproteins, and the Risk of Coronary Heart Disease." The Framingham Study, *Annals of Internal Medicine*, 74: 1–12, 1971.

Kannel, W.B., Castelli, W.P., and Gordon, T. "Cholesterol in the Prediction of Atherosclerotic Disease: New Perspectives on the Framingham Study." *Annals of Internal Medicine*, 90: 85–91, 1979.

Mann, G. V., "Diet—Heart: End of an Era," *New England Journal of Medicine*, 297:12, pp. 644–649, 1977.

Report of Inter-Society Commission for Heart Disease Resources. "Primary Prevention of Atherosclerotic Diseases." *Circulation,* Vol. XLII, December 1970, revised April 1972.

Stamler, J., "Epidemiology of Coronary Heart Disease," *Medical Clinics of North America*, 57:1, pp. 5–46, 1973.

Turpeinen, O., "Effect of Cholesterol-Lowering Diet on Mortality from Coronary Heart Disease and Other Causes," *Circulation* 59:1, pp. 1–7, 1979.

Abby G. Abelson, M.D., in Cleveland, Ohio, is a graduate of Case Western Reserve University School of Medicine.

RECOMMENDED DAILY DIETARY ALLOWANCES (RDA'S)*

Designed for the maintenance of good nutrition of practically all healthy persons in the U.S.A.

SEX/AGE CATEGORY	Years From	To	WEIGHT Pounds	HEIGHT Inches	FOOD ENERGY Calories
Children	1	3	29	35	1300
	4	6	44	44	1700
	7	10	62	52	2400
Males	11	14	99	62	2700
	15	18	145	69	2800
	19	22	154	70	2900
	23	50	154	70	2700
	51	75	154	70	2400
	76+		154	70	2050
Females	11	14	101	62	2200
	15	18	120	64	2100
	19	22	120	64	2100
	23	50	120	64	2000
	51	75	120	64	1800
	76+		120	64	1600
Pregnancy					+300
Lactation					+500

*The allowances are intended to provide for individual variations among most normal persons as they live in the United States under usual environmental stresses.

Reproduced from *Recommended Dietary Allowances*, Ninth Edition, (1980), with the permission of the National Academy of Sciences, Washington, D.C.

PART VIII

CALORIE COUNTER

The foods are listed according to the department in which they are found in the supermarket.

The number of calories is listed in the usual serving size, unless otherwise specified.

FRESH PRODUCE DEPARTMENT

Fresh Vegetables:

Calories are based on cooked vegetables, unless otherwise specified.

NAME	AMOUNT	CALORIES
Artichoke (med.)	1 bud	10–53*
Asparagus	4 spears	12
Beans, green	½ cup	17
Beans, lima	½ cup	95
Beans, yellow	½ cup	14
Beets	½ cup	27
Broccoli	½ cup	20
Brussels sprouts	½ cup	28
Cabbage (raw)	½ cup	9
Carrots	½ cup	24
Cauliflower	½ cup	14
Celery (raw)	½ cup	10
Collards	½ cup	21
Corn, ear	one ear	70
Cucumber (raw)	½ cup	10

*Calories range from 10 calories for freshly harvested artichokes to 53 calories for stored artichokes.

FRESH PRODUCE (continued)

NAME	AMOUNT	CALORIES
Eggplant	½ cup	19
Endive (raw)	½ cup	5
Garlic (raw)	1 clove	4
Green pepper (raw)	½ cup	9
Lettuce (raw)	½ cup	4
Mushrooms (raw)	½ cup	10
Onions	½ cup	31
Peas	½ cup	57
Potatoes	½ cup	59
Spinach	½ cup	21
Squash	½ cup	15
Sweet potatoes	½ cup	146
Swiss chard	½ cup	16
Tomatoes (med. raw)	one	27
Turnip	½ cup	18
Zucchini	½ cup	11

Fresh Fruits:

Calories are based on raw fruits.

Apple (med.)	one	61
Apricot (med.)	three	55
Avocado	one half	188
Banana (med.)	one	101
Blueberries	½ cup	45
Cantaloupe	one half	82
Cherries	½ cup	41
Coconut	½ cup	139
Cranberries	½ cup	22
Grapefruit	one half	40
Grapefruit juice	½ cup	48

Fresh Fruits (continued)

NAME	AMOUNT	CALORIES
Grapes	½ cup	35
Honeydew	wedge	49
Orange (med)	one	71
Orange juice	½ cup	66
Peach (med.)	one	38
Pear (med.)	one	86
Pineapple	½ cup	41
Plum (med.)	one	32
Raspberries (black)	½ cup	49
Raspberries (red)	½ cup	35
Rhubarb	½ cup	10
Strawberries	½ cup	28
Tangerine (med.)	one	39
Watermelon	¹⁄₁₆th of melon	111

Dried Fruits: (uncooked)

Apricots	½ cup	166
Dates	½ cup	311
Figs (med.)	one	40
Prunes (softened)	½ cup	230
Raisins	½ cup	210

Nuts: (shelled, unsalted)

Almonds	½ cup	425
Brazil	½ cup	458
Cashews	½ cup	393
Peanuts	½ cup	419
Pecans	½ cup	371
Walnuts (black, chopped)	½ cup	393
Walnuts (English, chopped)	½ cup	391

FRESH MEATS, POULTRY, FISH—PROCESSED MEATS

Calories are based on 4 oz. retail cuts, *cooked*.

Fresh Meats—Lean, Trimmed of Separable Fat

NAME	AMOUNT	CALORIES
Beef:		
Chuck arm	4 oz.	328
Club steak	4 oz.	277
Corned beef brisket	4 oz.	422
Flank	4 oz.	222
Ground chuck (21% fat)	4 oz.	324
Ground round (10% fat)	4 oz.	248
Plate (shortribs)	4 oz.	226
Porterhouse steak	4 oz.	254
Rib roast	4 oz.	273
Round steak	4 oz.	214
Rump roast	4 oz.	236
Sirloin steak	4 oz.	235
T-Bone steak	4 oz.	253
Lamb:		
Leg	4 oz.	211
Loin chops	4 oz.	213
Rib chops	4 oz.	240
Shoulder	4 oz.	233

Calories are based on 4 oz. retail cuts, *cooked*.

NAME	AMOUNT	CALORIES
Pork:		
Bacon (4 med. slices)	3.2 oz.	172
Bacon, Canadian (3 slices)	3 oz.	174
Boston butt	4 oz.	277
Ham, canned	4 oz.	219
Ham, fresh	4 oz.	246
Ham, light cure (smoked)	4 oz.	212
Loin	4 oz.	288
Picnic	4 oz.	241
Spareribs	4 oz.	499
Veal:		
Breast	4 oz.	344
Chuck	4 oz.	267
Leg	4 oz.	245
Loin	4 oz.	265
Rib	4 oz.	305
Organ Meats:		
Beef liver	1 slice	195
Brains	3 oz.	106
Calf liver	1 slice	222
Chicken liver	3 small	123
Heart	4 oz.	213
Kidneys (beef)	4 oz.	286
Sweetbreads	3 oz.	272
Sauerkraut	½ cup	21
Lard	1 Tbs.	117

FRESH MEATS, POULTRY, FISH—PROCESSED MEATS

NAME	AMOUNT	CALORIES
Poultry: (without skin; 4 oz. portion, cooked)		
Chicken—light meat	4 oz.	188
—dark meat	4 oz.	199
Turkey—light meat	4 oz.	199
—dark meat	4 oz.	230
Duck (roasted)	3 slices	310
Goose (roasted)	3 slices	322
Processed Meats:		
Beef, dried	3 oz.	174
Bologna, Lebanon	1 oz.	95*
Frankfurter (1 weiner)	2 oz.	176
Ham, chopped	1 oz.	65*
Ham, loaf	1 oz.	35*
Liverwurst	1¼ oz.	115*
Olive loaf	1 oz.	65*
Sausage (3 links)	3 oz.	186
Turkey roll	3.5 oz.	120*
Fish: (Raw-edible portions)		
Cod	4 oz.	89
Crab	4 oz.	98
Haddock	4 oz.	90
Halibut	4 oz.	114
Lobster (meat only)	4 oz.	69
Oysters	4 oz.	75
Perch	4 oz.	103
Pike	4 oz.	106
Salmon (sockeye)	4 oz.	136
Scallops	4 oz.	92
Shrimp	4 oz.	103
Snapper	4 oz.	106
Sole	4 oz.	90

*Data supplied by manufacturer.

DAIRY AND
REFRIGERATED PRODUCTS

NAME	AMOUNT	CALORIES
Butter (unsalted)	1 Tbs.	102
Butter, stick (salted)	1 Tbs.	102
Butter, whipped (salted)	1 Tbs.	68
Margarine, stick	1 Tbs.	102
Margarine, whipped, soft tub	1 Tbs.	68
Coffee cream (light)	1 Tbs.	29
Cream, half-and-half	1 Tbs.	20
Cream, heavy whipping	1 Tbs.	52
Cream, sour	1 Tbs.	26
Imitation sour cream (nondairy)	1 Tbs.	29
Whipped cream topping (pressurized)	1 Tbs.	8
Whole egg	one	79

Egg yolk is a concentrated source of cholesterol.

Milk:

Buttermilk, cultured	1 cup	99
Skim milk	1 cup	86
Low-fat milk, 2% fat	1 cup	121
Low-fat milk, 1% fat	1 cup	102
Whole milk, 3.3% fat	1 cup	150
Whole milk, 3.7% fat	1 cup	157
Chocolate milk (from low-fat 1% milk)	1 cup	158
Chocolate milk (from low-fat 2% milk)	1 cup	179
Chocolate milk (from whole milk)	1 cup	208
Eggnog	1 cup	342
Yogurt, plain—low-fat	1 cup	144
Yogurt, fruit-flavored	1 cup	231

DAIRY AND REFRIGERATED PRODUCTS

NAME	AMOUNT	CALORIES
Cheese:		
American, pasteurized	1 oz.	93
Brick	1 oz.	105
Blue	1 oz.	100
Camembert	1 oz.	85
Cheddar	1 oz.	114
Colby	1 oz.	112
Cottage cheese, creamed	½ cup	117
Cottage cheese, dry	½ cup	96
Cottage cheese, low-fat 1%	½ cup	82
Cottage cheese, low-fat 2%	½ cup	101
Cream cheese	1 oz.	99
Edam	1 oz.	101
Feta	1 oz.	75
Gouda	1 oz.	101
Gruyère	1 oz.	117
Monterey Jack	1 oz.	106
Mozzarella, low-moisture part-skim	1 oz.	79
Neufchatel	1 oz.	74
Parmesan	1 oz.	129
Ricotta (part-skim)	½ cup	171
Roquefort	1 oz.	105
Skim-milk cheese spread (processed) (less than 5% fat)	1 oz.	35
Swiss, pasteurized	1 oz.	95
Refrigerated Products:		
Horseradish	1 Tbs.	6
Herring (pickled)	½ cup	252
Dill pickles	1 lg.	15
Refrigerated cookie dough	3 oz.	449
Smoked salmon	2 oz.	100

FROZEN FOODS

NAME	AMOUNT	CALORIES
Frozen Fruits and Fruit Juices:		
Blackberries	½ cup	46
Blueberries	½ cup	46
Cherries, red sour	½ cup	62
Grape juice	½ cup	66
Grapefruit juice (unsweetened)	½ cup	51
Honeydew melon balls	½ cup	72
Lemonade concentrate*	½ cup	54
Limeade concentrate*	½ cup	51
Orange juice concentrate*	½ cup	61
Raspberries, red	½ cup	123
Rhubarb	½ cup	85
Strawberries	½ cup	139
Frozen Vegetables: (Cooked)		
Asparagus	½ cup	22
Broccoli	½ cup	24
Brussels sprouts	½ cup	26
Cauliflower	½ cup	16
Corn, kernels	½ cup	68
Corn, ear	one med.	122
Green beans	½ cup	17
Lima beans	½ cup	82
Mixed vegetables	½ cup	74
Peas	½ cup	54
Potatoes, raw (diced or shredded)	½ cup	51
Potatoes, raw (french fried)	10 pcs.	111
Spinach, chopped	½ cup	24
Squash, winter	½ cup	46
Succotash	½ cup	75
Yellow beans	½ cup	18

*diluted

FROZEN FOODS

NAME	AMOUNT	CALORIES
Frozen Vegetables: (in sauces or breaded)		
Corn fritters	4 oz.	260*
Creamed spinach	3 oz.	60*
Fried eggplant	3.5 oz.	260*
Glazed carrots	3.3 oz.	80*
Glazed sweet potatoes	4 oz.	180*
Potato balls, breaded	2.5 oz.	190*
Frozen Fish and Shellfish:		
Fried Perch	4 oz.	250*
Fried Shrimp	3 oz.	170*
Frozen Poultry:		
Frozen turkey, butter-basted (white meat only)	3.5 oz.	170*
Frozen turkey roll	3.5 oz.	120*

Frozen Dinners: (one complete dinner)

Frozen dinners are not color-coded because the saturated fat/cholesterol content varies widely among manufacturers.

NAME	AMOUNT	CALORIES
Beans and franks	11¼ oz.	550*
Beef	11½ oz.	370*
Beef pot pie	8 oz.	430*
Chicken and noodles	10¼ oz.	390*
Chicken pot pie	8 oz.	450*
Chopped sirloin	10 oz.	460*
Fish n' chips	10¼ oz.	450*
Fried chicken	11½ oz.	570*
Ham	10¼ oz.	380*
Macaroni and beef	12 oz.	400*
Spaghetti and meatballs	12½ oz.	410*
Swiss steak	10 oz.	350*
Turkey	11½ oz.	360*
Veal parmigiana	12¼ oz.	520*

*Data supplied by manufacturers.

FROZEN FOODS

NAME	AMOUNT	CALORIES
Egg substitutes	¼ cup	70–80*
Coffee whitener (nondairy)	1 Tbs.	20
Dessert topping (nondairy), pressurized	1 Tbs.	11
Dessert topping (nondairy), semisolid	1 Tbs.	13
Frozen Bakery:		
Blueberry muffin	one	120*
Corn muffin	one	130*
Croissant	one	109*
Parkerhouse roll	one	75*
Poppy seed roll	one	55*
Sesame seed roll	one	55*
Doughnut, glazed	one	150*
Doughnut, jelly	one	180*
Apple pie	⅙ pie	231
Cherry pie	⅙ pie	282
Coconut cream pie	⅙ pie	249
Banana cake	⅛ cake	175*
Chocolate brownie	⅛ cake	200*
Devil's food cake	⅙ cake	323
Frozen pizza (5″ indiv.)	one	178
Waffle (plain, 1¼ oz.)	one	86
Waffle (egg, 1¼ oz.)	one	120*

*Data supplied by manufacturer.

CEREALS AND TOASTER PASTRIES

Calorie content for hot cereals has been taken directly from the nutrition information on the package label.

The hot and cold cereals are not color-coded because the color-coding would depend on the fat content of the milk added to the cereal—whole, lowfat, or skim.

NAME	AMOUNT	CALORIES
Hot Cereals: (uncooked, without added milk)		
Cream of Rice	¾ cup**	120
Cream of Wheat (Regular)	1 oz.	100
Cream of Wheat (Instant)	1 oz.	100
Cream of Wheat (Quick)	1 oz.	100
Cream of Wheat (Mix-N-Eat)	1 oz.	100
Cream of Wheat (Mix-N-Eat) maple flavor	1¼ oz.	130
Malt-O-Meal (Quick)	1 oz.	100
Maypo (30-second)	1 oz.	110
Quaker Hot and Creamy	1 oz.	101
Quaker Whole Wheat	1 oz.	100
Quaker Oatmeal (Old Fashioned)	1 oz.	109
Quaker Oatmeal (Quick)	1 oz.	109
Ralston (Regular)	1 oz.	110
Wheatena	1 oz.	110

Ready-to-Eat Cereals

Since calorie content on ready-to-eat cereals varies among manufacturers, the figures for calories have been taken from the *United States Department of Agriculture Handbook* No. 456.

Bran Cereal Products:

Bran flakes (40%)	1 cup	106
Bran flakes with raisins	1 cup	144

**Cooked serving.

CEREALS AND TOASTER PASTRIES

NAME	AMOUNT	CALORIES
Bran Cereal Products: (continued)		
Bran with wheat germ	2 Tbs.	22
Bran with malt extract	2 Tbs.	18
Corn Cereal Products:		
Cornflakes	1 cup	97
Sugar-coated cornflakes	1 cup	154
Puffed corn	1 cup	80
Cocoa-flavored corn	1 cup	117
Fruit-flavored corn	1 cup	119
Oat Cereal Products:		
Shredded oats with sugar	1 cup	171
Puffed oats with sugar	1 cup	99
Puffed oats with corn	1 cup	139
Rice Cereal Products:		
Puffed rice	1 cup	60
Puffed rice with cocoa	1 cup	140
Oven popped with sugar	1 cup	117
Shredded rice with sugar	1 cup	98
Wheat Cereal Products:		
Wheat, puffed (plain)	1 cup	54
Wheat, puffed with sugar	1 cup	132
Wheat and malted barley (flakes)	1 cup	157
Wheat and malted barley (granules)	½ cup	215

CEREALS AND TOASTER PASTRIES

NAME	AMOUNT	CALORIES
Wheatflakes with sugar	1 cup	106
Wheat germ (plain)	1 Tbs.	23
Shredded wheat	1 biscuit	89
Shredded wheat, spoon size, (50 small)	1 cup	177
"Natural" cereals	1 oz.	130*
Breakfast bars	1 bar	200*
Cornmeal (enriched)	1 cup	502
Cornmeal (self-rising)	1 cup	465

Toaster Pastries:

Plain: (one pastry)

Blueberry	one	210*
Brown sugar-cinnamon	one	210*
Strawberry	one	210*
Raspberry	one	210*

Frosted: (one pastry)

Blueberry	one	210*
Brown sugar-cinnamon	one	210*
Strawberry	one	210*
Raspberry	one	210*

*Data supplied by manufacturer.

CANNED FOODS

NAME	AMOUNT	CALORIES
Fruits and Fruit Juices:		
Apple juice	½ cup	59
Apple sauce	½ cup	50
Apricots (heavy syrup)	½ cup	111
Apricot nectar	½ cup	72
Blackberries	½ cup	117
Cherries (heavy syrup)	½ cup	104
Cherries (sour)	½ cup	53
Cranberry juice	½ cup	82
Cranberry sauce	½ cup	202
Figs	½ cup	109
Fruit cocktail	½ cup	97
Grape drink	½ cup	68
Grape juice	½ cup	84
Grapefruit sections	½ cup	89
Grapefruit juice	½ cup	52
Orange juice	½ cup	60
Peaches (heavy syrup)	½ cup	100
Pears (heavy syrup)	½ cup	97
Pineapple (in its own juice)	½ cup	48
Pineapple (heavy syrup)	½ cup	117
Pineapple juice	½ cup	69
Plums (heavy syrup)	½ cup	107
Prune juice	½ cup	99
Pumpkin	½ cup	40

CANNED FOODS (continued)

NAME	AMOUNT	CALORIES
Canned Vegetables (drained solids) and		
Vegetable Juices:		
Asparagus	½ cup	26
Beans, green	½ cup	16
Beans, lima	½ cup	82
Beans, yellow	½ cup	23
Beets (sliced)	½ cup	32
Carrots	½ cup	24
Corn, whole kernel	½ cup	87
Corn, cream style	½ cup	105
Mushrooms	½ cup	18
Peas	½ cup	75
Sauerkraut	½ cup	21
Spinach	½ cup	25
Sweet potatoes	½ cup	108
Tomatoes (solids and liquids)	½ cup	26
Tomato juice	½ cup	23
Vegetable juice cocktail	½ cup	21

Soups: (canned, prepared with equal amounts of water)

NAME	AMOUNT	CALORIES
Beef noodle	1 cup	67
Chicken noodle	1 cup	62
Chicken rice	1 cup	48
Cream of chicken	1 cup	94
Manhattan clam chowder	1 cup	81
Minestrone	1 cup	105
Onion	1 cup	65
Pea	1 cup	130

NAME	AMOUNT	CALORIES
Soups: (continued)		
Tomato	1 cup	88
Turkey noodle	1 cup	79
Vegetarian vegetable	1 cup	78
Vegetable beef	1 cup	78

Soups: (canned, prepared with equal amounts of milk)

Cream of celery	1 cup	169
Cream of chicken	1 cup	179
Cream of mushroom	1 cup	216
Tomato	1 cup	173
Pea	1 cup	213

Soups: Dehydrated (prepared as directed on package)

Beef noodle	1 cup	67
Bouillon cube	one	5
Chicken noodle	1 cup	53
Onion	1 cup	36
Tomato-vegetable	1 cup	65

Canned Fish:

Crabmeat	¼ cup	34
Salmon (pink)	½ cup	160
Salmon (red, sockeye)	½ cup	194
Sardines (in oil)	3¾ oz. can	330
Shrimp	20 small	152
Tuna fish (water pack)	3½ oz. can	126

CANNED FOODS (continued)

NAME	AMOUNT	CALORIES
Ready-to-Serve Main Dishes:		
Beans and franks	1 cup	367
Baked beans in tomato		
sauce	1 cup	306
Chili con carne	1 cup	339
Macaroni and cheese	1 cup	228
Pork and beans	1 cup	311
Processed canned meats:		
Pork, chopped		
(spiced/unspiced)	2 oz.	167
Pork sausage	2 patties	299
Vienna sausage	2 oz.	127
Spaghetti and meatballs	1 cup	258
Spaghetti, tomato sauce		
with cheese	1 cup	190
Vegetable and beef stew	1 cup	194
Chinese Foods:		
Chop suey with meat	8 oz.	141
Chow mein with chicken	8 oz.	86
Soy sauce	1 Tbs.	12

Calorie contents of tomato paste, tomato puree, and spaghetti sauces are listed on page 115.

CAKE AND PIE MIXES, DESSERTS, BAKING AIDS

The serving size of some products in this department is figured for a whole recipe, rather than a usual serving. Note the serving size when checking calorie content on a particular food.

NAME	AMOUNT	CALORIES
Cake flour (enriched)*	1 cup	430
Bread flour (enriched)*	1 cup	420
All-purpose flour (enriched)*	1 cup	455
Self-rising flour (enriched)*	1 cup	405
Whole wheat flour	1 cup	400
Biscuit mix (dry) (enriched flour)	½ cup	255
Graham cracker crumbs for piecrusts	1 cup	432
Piecrust mix	10 oz. pkg.	1482
Roll mix (water)	one roll	105
Sugars:		
Brown	1 cup	821
Confectioners	1 cup	462
White granulated	1 cup	770
Syrups:		
Maple syrup	1 Tbs.	50
Molasses (light)	1 Tbs.	50
Molasses (blackstrap)	1 Tbs.	43
Pancake syrup (corn blend)	1 Tbs.	59

---

*"Enriched" means that vitamins have been added.

CAKE AND PIE MIXES, DESSERTS, BAKING AIDS

NAME	AMOUNT	CALORIES
Cakes: (made from baking mix); one piece		
Angel food	¹⁄₁₂ of whole	137
Brownies	one	86
Chocolate cake	¹⁄₁₂ of whole	308
Coffee cake	¹⁄₆ of whole	232
Devil's food cake	¹⁄₁₂ of whole	312
Honey spice cake	¹⁄₁₂ of whole	363
White cake	¹⁄₁₂ of whole	333
Yellow cake	¹⁄₁₂ of whole	310
Corn muffin mix	one muffin	130
Cornbread mix	one piece	178
Pancake and waffle mix (dry)	½ cup	262
Frosting:		
Chocolate fudge	¼ cup	293
Creamy fudge	¼ cup	208
"Light" frosting mix (white)	¹⁄₁₂ of pkg.	60*
(chocolate)	¹⁄₁₂ of pkg.	100*
Powdered dessert topping (nondairy)	1 Tbs.	8*

*Data supplied by manufacturer.

CAKE AND PIE MIXES, DESSERTS, BAKING AIDS

NAME	AMOUNT	CALORIES
Milk, condensed, sweetened	¼ cup	246
Milk, evaporated, skim	¼ cup	50
Milk, evaporated, whole	¼ cup	85
Nonfat dry milk, instant	8 fl. oz.**	80

Baking Aids:

Baking soda	1 tsp.	0
Baking powder	1 tsp.	4
Chocolate (baking, bitter)	1 oz.	143
Chocolate (semisweet morsels)	1 oz.	144
Cornstarch	1 tsp.	29
Coconut (shredded)	½ cup	139
Salt	1 tsp.	0
Tapioca (dry)	1 Tbs.	30
Vegetable shortening (solid)	1 Tbs.	111

Gelatins: (prepared as directed on package)

Gelatin, unflavored, dry	1 Tbs.	34

Gelatin, flavored:
Apricot, blackberry, black cherry, black raspberry, cherry, concord grape, mixed fruit, orange, peach, raspberry, strawberry, strawberry-banana, wild cherry, wild raspberry.

	½ cup	80*

---

*Data supplied by manufacturer.
**Reconstituted

CAKE AND PIE MIXES, DESSERTS, BAKING AIDS

NAME	AMOUNT	CALORIES
Puddings: (prepared as directed on package)		
Tapioca pudding, chocolate	½ cup	160*
Tapioca pudding, vanilla	½ cup	160*
Rice pudding	½ cup	170*
Pudding and pie filling: (regular)		
Butterscotch	½ cup	170*
Chocolate	½ cup	170*
Vanilla	½ cup	160*
Banana cream	⅙ of 8" pie	110*
Coconut cream	⅙ of 9" pie	110*
Lemon	⅙ of 9" pie	180*
Pudding and pie filling: (instant)		
Banana cream	½ cup	180*
Butterscotch	½ cup	170*
Chocolate	½ cup	190*
Coconut cream	½ cup	180*
Lemon	½ cup	180*
Pistachio	½ cup	180*
Vanilla	½ cup	180*

*Data supplied by manufacturer.

SPAGHETTI, NOODLES, RICE, BEANS, SAUCES

NAME	AMOUNT	CALORIES
Gravy Mixes: (prepared as directed on package)		
Au jus gravy mix	¼ cup	8*
Brown gravy mix	¼ cup	15*
Cheese sauce mix	¼ cup	84*
Chicken gravy mix	¼ cup	22*
Hollandaise sauce	¼ cup	58*
Mushroom gravy mix	¼ cup	15*
Onion gravy mix	¼ cup	21*
Turkey gravy mix	¼ cup	23*
Beans: (dried)		
Barley, pearled	½ cup	348
Great northern or navy	½ cup	306
Dried chickpeas	½ cup	360
Dried peas	½ cup	340
Dried kidney beans	½ cup	317
Dried lentils	½ cup	323
Dried lima beans	½ cup	310
Dried pinto beans	½ cup	332
Noodles, Pasta: (cooked)		
Macaroni	½ cup	96
Noodles, egg	½ cup	100
Spaghetti, plain	½ cup	78
Rice: (cooked, prepared as directed on package)		
Brown	½ cup	116
Flavored rice mix	½ cup	120*
Instant	½ cup	90
Spanish rice mix	½ cup	100*
White long grain	½ cup	112

*Data supplied by manufacturer.

SPAGHETTI, NOODLES, RICE, BEANS, SAUCES

NAME	AMOUNT	CALORIES
Bottled or Canned Sauces:		
Meatless spaghetti sauce (bottled)	4 oz.	70*
Spaghetti sauce with meat (bottled)	4 oz.	100*
Tomato paste	2 oz.	50*
Tomato puree	4 oz.	50*
Tomato sauce	4 oz.	40*
Potatoes: (cooked, prepared as directed on package)		
Dehydrated mashed flakes	½ cup	98
Dehydrated mashed granules	½ cup	83
Dehydrated potatoes au gratin	½ cup	90*
Dehydrated potatoes, creamed	½ cup	90*
Pizza Mixes:		
Pizza mix	3½ oz.	200*
Cheese pizza mix	3¾ oz.	220*
Hamburger pizza mix	4¼ oz.	300*
Pepperoni pizza mix	4¼ oz.	270*
Sausage pizza mix	4¼ oz.	280*

---

*Data supplied by manufacturer.

SALAD DRESSINGS, OLIVES, PICKLES, OILS

NAME	AMOUNT	CALORIES
Cooking Oils:		
Corn, cottonseed, safflower, sesame, soybean, sunflower, or blend	1 Tbs.	120
Peanut oil	1 Tbs.	119
Olive oil	1 Tbs.	119
Olives and Pickles:		
Green olives (large)	five	23
Ripe olives (mammoth)	five	36
Pickles, dill (med.)	one	7
Pickle relish	1 Tbs.	21
All vinegars	1 Tbs.	2
Bacon bits, imitation	1 tsp.	8*
Salad Dressings: (bottled)		
Blue, Roquefort	1 Tbs.	76
French	1 Tbs.	66
Italian	1 Tbs.	83
Thousand Island	1 Tbs.	80
Mayonnaise	1 Tbs.	101
Mayonnaise-type dressing	1 Tbs.	65
Salad Dressings: (dry mix)		
French creamy	1 Tbs.	70*
Italian	1 Tbs.	60*
Condiments:		
Barbecue sauce	1 Tbs.	14
Chili sauce	1 Tbs.	16
Mustard, prepared	1 Tbs.	12
Tomato ketchup	1 Tbs.	16
Worcestershire sauce	1 Tbs.	12

*Data supplied by manufacturer.

PACKAGED BAKERY: BREAD, ROLLS, CAKES, AND PIES—COOKIES AND CRACKERS

NAME	AMOUNT	CALORIES
Breads:		
Cracked wheat	1 slice	66
French or Vienna	1 slice	73
Italian	1 slice	83
Pumpernickel	1 slice	79
Raisin	1 slice	66
Rye or whole wheat	1 slice	61
White enriched	1 slice	68
Pita bread	1 piece	200
Rolls:		
Brown and serve	1 roll	84
Cloverleaf	1 roll	83
English muffin	one	130*
Frankfurter, hamburger	1 roll	119
Kaiser	1 roll	156
Bread Products:		
Bread crumbs (plain)	2 Tbs.	49
Bread sticks	one	106
Bread stuffing (dry)	¼ cup	65
Corn flake crumbs	2 Tbs.	41
Herb seasoned croutons	2 Tbs.	50*
Matzo (unsalted)	1 piece	78
Melba toast (unsalted)	1 piece	15
Cakes, Pies, Doughnuts, Danish:		
Cupcakes (chocolate)	one	160*
Cakes, filled, miniature	one	140*
Danish pastry, 4″ × 1″	one	274
Doughnut, plain (1½ oz.)	one	164
Pies: (individual)		
Apple	4½ oz.	400*
Cherry	4½ oz.	420*

*Data supplied by manufacturer.

PACKAGED BAKERY: BREAD, ROLLS, CAKES, PIES—COOKIES AND CRACKERS

NAME	AMOUNT	CALORIES
Cookies:		
Brownie	one	103
Butter wafer	one	23
Chocolate chip	one	50
Coconut bar	one	45
Fig bar	one	50
Ginger snap	one	29
Graham cracker, chocolate covered	one	62
Lady finger	one	40
Macaroon	one	91
Marshmallow	one	73
Molasses	one	137
Oatmeal raisin	one	59
Sandwich, chocolate or vanilla	one	50
Sugar wafer	one	46
Vanilla wafer	one	19
Crackers:		
Butter cracker	one	15
Cheese cracker	one	15
Graham cracker (plain)	one	55
Graham cracker (sugar honey)	one	58
Rye wafer (whole grain)	one	22
Saltine	one	12
Soda cracker	one	22
Zwieback	one	30

JELLIES, ICE CREAM, CANDY, SYRUPS

NAME	AMOUNT	CALORIES
Jellies:		
Jellies	1 Tbs.	49
Apple butter	1 Tbs.	33
Honey	1 Tbs.	64
Jams and preserves	1 Tbs.	54
Orange marmalade	1 Tbs.	51
Peanut butter	1 Tbs.	94
Ice Cream Products:		
Ice cream (16% fat)	½ cup	165
Ice cream (10% fat)	½ cup	129
Ice milk	½ cup	100
Orange sherbet	½ cup	130
Candy:		
Butterscotch	1 oz.	113
Candy corn	1 oz.	103
Caramel	1 oz.	113
Chocolate caramel	1 oz.	121
Chocolate fudge	1 oz.	122
Chocolate (milk with almonds)	1 oz.	151
Chocolate (milk with peanuts)	1 oz.	154
Chocolate (semisweet)	1 oz.	150
Chocolate-covered raisins	1 oz.	120
Cream mints	1 oz.	116
Gum drops	1 oz.	98
Hard candy	1 oz.	109
Jelly beans	1 oz.	104
Marshmallow	1 oz.	23
Syrups:		
Butterscotch sauce	1 oz.	203
Chocolate syrup (thin)	1 oz.	92
Chocolate syrup (fudge)	1 oz.	124

SNACKS—BEVERAGES

NAME	AMOUNT	CALORIES
Caramel corn	1 cup	134
Cheese puffs	1 oz.	160*
Cheese snack crackers	10	150
Corn chips	1 oz.	170*
Popcorn	1 cup	41
Potato chips	10 chips	114
Pretzels (thin type)	10	234
Nuts:		
Almonds (unsalted)	9–10 nuts	60
Cashews (unsalted)	7 nuts	80
Peanuts (salted) Spanish	1 oz.	166
Pecans (unsalted)	10 halves	62
Soy nuts	1 oz.	130*
Sunflower seeds (unsalted)	1 oz.	102
Beverages:		
Club soda	8 oz.	0*
Coca-Cola	8 oz.	104
Ginger-ale	8 oz.	80
Cocoa, dry powder	1 Tbs.	14
Cocoa mix hot (prepared)	1 oz.	120*
Coffee, dry powder	1 Tbs.	3
Coffee, flavored, powder (prepared)	6 oz.	50–60*
Coffee whitener (powdered) (nondairy)	1 tsp.	11
Wine, cooking	2 oz.	19*
Wine, dessert	3½ oz.	141
Wine, table	3½ oz.	87
Chocolate instant drink mix	3 tsp.	70*
Strawberry instant drink mix	3 tsp.	80*

*Data supplied by manufacturer.

PART IX

WHY THIS BOOK WAS WRITTEN

As a nutritionist and author of two cookbooks, Janet James was often asked for help with special health problems related to foods. She was frequently asked questions like the following:

"My doctor says I have to cut down on fat and cholesterol in my diet—can you tell me the foods that I *can* eat?"

"Do I have to give up my favorite fast-food lunch? Is there anything I can eat at a restaurant that's low in fat?"

To fully answer these questions, Ms. James knew that she needed to research the fat and cholesterol contents of all the foods in the American diet. She realized that this would be a long and difficult task, and so she asked Lois Goulder for help.

Together they began a search that led them to many experts. For assistance with the Supermarket-Shopping Guide, they consulted Helen B. Brown, Ph.D., Research Consultant and Nutritionist at the Cleveland Clinic. She has been consultant for the National Heart, Lung, and Blood Institute and the U.S. Department of Agriculture.

They also consulted with university nutritionists, food editors, nurses, and hospital dietitians. Physicians were consulted for information relating fat/cholesterol intake to coronary heart disease.

They turned to the Department of Agriculture for their latest data. Food manufacturers were consulted for information on the fat/cholesterol contents of their products. The leading fast-food restaurant chains were contacted for their latest nutritional information.

After completing their research, they knew that the extensive material they had compiled would be of invaluable help to anyone wanting to cut down on saturated fat/cholesterol. The result is the DELL COLOR-CODED LOW-FAT-LIVING GUIDE.

BIBLIOGRAPHY

CHOLESTEROL CONTENT OF FOODS. Feeley, Ruth M., Patricia E. Criner, and Bernice K. Watt, Consumer and Food Economics, Research Division, Agricultural Research Service, U.S. Department of Agriculture, Hyattsville, Maryland, *Journal of the American Dietetic Association,* Vol. 61, no. 2, August 1972.

COMPOSITION OF FOODS—Dairy and Egg Products: Raw, Processed, Prepared. Agriculture Handbook No. 8-1. United States Department of Agriculture, Washington, D.C., revised November 1976.

COMPOSITION OF FOODS—Raw, Processed, Prepared. Agriculture Handbook No. 8. United States Department of Agriculture, Washington, D.C., October 1975.

COMPOSITION OF FOODS—Spices and Herbs: Raw, Processed, Prepared Agriculture Handbook No. 8-2. United States Department of Agriculture, Washington, D.C., revised January 1977.

CURRENT FOCUS ON FAT IN THE DIET. Brown, Helen B., Ph.D. White Paper, The American Dietetic Association, 1977

DIETARY GOALS FOR THE UNITED STATES Second Edition. Select Committee on Nutrition and Human Needs, United States Senate. U.S. Government Printing Office, Washington, D.C., December 1977.

FOOD VALUES OF PORTIONS COMMONLY USED. Bowes and Church, Twelfth Edition. Revised by Charles F. Church, Helen N. Church. J.B. Lippincott Co., Philadelphia, 1975.

NUTRITIVE VALUE OF AMERICAN FOODS. Adams, Catherine F. In Common Units. Agriculture Handbook No. 456. United States Department of Agriculture, Washington, D.C., issued November 1975.

The fat and cholesterol content of some foods has been supplied by manufacturers, or taken directly from nutrition information printed on the prodduct label.

The Calorie-Activity Chart was based on information from:

Obesity in Perspective, Department of Health, Education and Welfare, Publication No. NIH 75:708, National Institute of Health, Bethesda, Maryland, 1973.

About the Authors

A graduate of the Department of Nutrition of Case Western Reserve University, Janet James is well known in the northern Ohio area as a popular lecturer and demonstrator on easy-to-prepare gourmet foods.

As former head of the consumer services division of a major supermarket chain, she became aware of the special diet needs of many consumers. She is co-author of *Better Meals for YOU with Low-Calorie Gourmet Recipes*, endorsed by the Greater Cleveland Diabetic Association. Her first book, *Quick Cuisine* was the result of her simple adaptations of authentic recipes from outstanding European chefs.

Lois Goulder did her undergraduate work at Cornell University and the Northwestern University School of Journalism, and later received her Master's Degree in Education at Case Western Reserve University.

Her work experience was in the fields of advertising public relations, education, and social service. Ms. Goulder's research skills and expertise in analyzing data were invaluable in organizing the vast amount of technical nutritional information that the authors compiled while writing these books: *THE DELL COLOR-CODED GUIDE TO LOW-SALT-LIVING,* and *THE DELL COLOR-CODED GUIDE TO LOW-FAT-LIVING.*

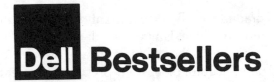

Dell Bestsellers

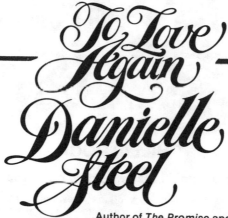

THE PASSING BELLS

by
PHILLIP ROCK

A story you'll wish would go on forever.

Here is the vivid story of the Grevilles, a titled British family, and their servants—men and women who knew their place, upstairs and down, until England went to war and the whole fabric of British society began to unravel and change.

"Well-written, exciting. Echoes of Hemingway, Graves and *Upstairs, Downstairs.*"—*Library Journal*

"Every twenty-five years or so, we are blessed with a war novel, outstanding in that it depicts not only the history of a time but also its soul."—*West Coast Review of Books.*

"Vivid and enthralling."—*The Philadelphia Inquirer*

A Dell Book $2.75   (16837-6)

At your local bookstore or use this handy coupon for ordering: